"Chorus of Souls offers sage advice from an inspired and compassionate teacher! Author Sheila Burke, shares her understanding of soul consciousness, synchronicity, and probes one of the most potent questions mankind can ask – what is the purpose of my life? Graciously written, Chorus of Souls leads us on a journey to better understanding the relationship between our soulful selves and the purposeful human beings we were born to be – a journey not to be missed!"
- **Heather McCloskey Beck**, author of *Take the Leap*

"When a truth comes to you, no matter what form, you feel a vibration start from deep within. This vibration gets stronger and stronger the more you delve into this truth, until it breaks free causing a light to shine forth from your eyes, your hands tingle at its power and you feel the shift within. You embrace this truth, you make it a part of your soul. Then you bring it out into the world with you. This is the amazing feeling I had from page one of Chorus of Souls. A truth which resonated to my very core. A book that made my soul sigh in contentment. I shall never be the same."
- **J.V. Manning**, author of *Random Thoughts n Lotsa Coffee*

"Life is a journey, and Sheila Burke explains how to make the most of that journey from the inside out. Perceptive and practical, "Chorus of Souls" is a marvelous work packed with thoughtful insights and life-changing wisdom we can all use for cultivating a healthy spirit!"
- **Patricia Saxton**, author and illustrator of *52 Weeks of Peace, A Book of Fairies, and The Book of Mermaids*

Chorus of Souls

Chorus of Souls

The Sacred Guide to Harmony, Healing, and Happiness

Sheila M. Burke

Om Sweet Om Publishing

Seven Hills, Ohio

sheilamburke.com

Om Sweet Om Publishing

Copyright © 2014 Sheila M. Burke
Published January 23, 2014
Printed and bound in the United States

Cover design by Sheila M. Burke © 2013
All photographs © Sheila M. Burke

ISBN-13: 978-0615898346 (Om Sweet Om)
ISBN-10: 0615898343
Library of Congress Card Number – Pending
Chorus of Souls: The Sacred Guide to Harmony, Healing, and
Happiness/ Sheila M. Burke ISBN-13: 978-0615898346 /
ISBN-10: 0615898343   Om Sweet Om Publishing

1st Edition

Dedication

Chorus of Souls is dedicated to each and every soul I have crossed paths with in this lifetime. I'm grateful for the love, and I'm even grateful for any hurt, for I have learned something from each and every one of you.

Table of Contents

Author's Acknowledgments

I wish to thank my husband Shane for being my partner for the last twenty five years. I am grateful for the experience of being able to journey together, whether it's our daily soul chats, nights filled with laughter, or working out the kinks. I'm blessed to have found you in this lifetime, and I'm looking forward to the next twenty five years.

To my children Kaylee, Kelsey, and Alan who completely amaze me every day. Thankfully we raised you to love and respect yourselves – we all know now that is the foundation for a healthy soul.

To Robin Renner my Editor-In-Chief and fellow soul sister: First it was "Zebra," now it's "Supa-script!"

Thank you to all my friends and family for your support over the years as I worked through life. I'd like to give a shout out to my Home Fry, Donna Algeri. Thanks to all my fellow members in the Inspiration Page Owners Group for all your love and support. We have come a long way over the years and have become one amazing and cohesive group of souls! Last but certainly not least, a special thank you to my friend and beautiful soul Laurel Bleadon-Maffei, of Illuminating Souls, who inspired the idea for this book during our long chats about soul family.

Introduction

The chorus is the most important part of a song. Repeating itself over and over again, the chorus carries the main theme and is most remembered. Our soul (our pure consciousness) *is our chorus.* It is the most powerful area of our structure, repeating itself over and over again. Not unlike the chorus of a song, the soul consciousness carries our message and expresses our main theme in the life we are here to live.

Chorus of Souls is a guide to awakening the authentic self by using the tools nestled deep within each of us. These tools, this sacred knowledge which each of us arrived here with, remain dormant until we are ready to awaken our spirit. Meet the chorus of souls and learn how we are interconnected, why we sometimes have that uncanny feeling that we've met someone before. Learn how to cultivate your own healthy spiritual practice and live a harmonious and happy life.

Chorus of Souls is also a guide to heal a sick soul. From time to time we all experience a sick soul, when we find ourselves out of sorts, seemingly wandering aimlessly. Like everyone else, I have experienced soul sickness a few times in my life. The important thing to remember is we all have the tools within ourselves to heal our soul and to live life as we were meant to – in harmony and happiness.

I am well aware of the outward appearing differences many people see in each other, and I have made it my goal to bring everything I've learned about spirit and pure consciousness into an easy to understand format in order to dispel those differences. Throughout this book I will reference God, The Divine, Universe, or a Higher Power, as *Source*. This is intentional as there are many beliefs and many names, but each name and every belief points us in the same direction in the end game. Awakening is not about changing your religion it is about living a healthy *spiritual* life. Chorus of Souls is my interpretation of my belief that *we are one*. I invite you to take away all that resonates with you.

Sacred and ancient knowledge transform within these pages into a clear and concise road map for the reader to take along on their journey of transformation. Life's important questions will be answered, and the answers may be simpler than you thought.

Welcome to the Chorus of Souls,
Sheila Burke

1.

Rise and Shine Sleepyhead!

Millions of people from every nook and cranny on this beautiful Earth have been captivated by the feeling of a great, big, full body stretch and are rubbing the sleep from their eyes. Happening for decades, we are now seeing a cosmic burst in the numbers of those experiencing this shift of consciousness. Humanity can feel something happening universally; the time has come where something wonderful and tremendous is bubbling up from the depths of our core – it is the essence of our own true spirit. We ask questions of ourselves such as *Who Am I? Why Am I here? Where Am I Going?* It is the beginning of our awakening. This book will help you answer these questions.

Awakening is not about religion. Awakening is the finding of the sacred within yourself; awakening is discovering your spirit; it is a day-by-day communication with your sacred self. See the beauty of yourself within, recognize the divine beauty of others with all inclination of personality aside. Find gratefulness and appreciation for all that is – simply because it is. Surrender personality and ego in order to live through spirit. Nourishing your spirit, strengthens your spirit and makes it healthy. A healthy spirit is able to comfort other spirits. See others as spirit rather than personality. That sole act will change your entire line of thinking.

The concepts of interconnectedness (We Are One), and that our consciousness is born of the Divine (and exist endlessly) – are Universal Spiritual Truths. Spiritual awareness is recognizing these spiritual truths and being mindful of the roles they play. Awakening, however, is actively living and understanding these truths. Spiritual awakening begins when you experience a sudden shift of consciousness and (the awakening) continues as your consciousness expands. As if a light switch has been flipped on after walking around a dark room, those who are awakening can now see life around them clearly. Focus shifts from ego based to Essence based. The shift can be small or big. Expansion of consciousness can increase over time, but if not nurtured can also decrease.

As we grow older spiritually we learn to tap into a space rooted deeply within us, and it becomes clear that we are all here for some greater purpose. Our physical body is merely a shell, a vehicle in which our soul travels in during its time here on Earth, and we are now beginning to understand how incredibly powerful the soul is in commandeering that vehicle.

Spiritual awakening is taking place all over the world. Some people might feel like a change is happening to them, but they cannot quite figure out what the change is. There are many signs of the awakening of spirit, which include: being more aware of your place on the Earth and within the Universe, feeling more connected, part of the larger whole, and being more attuned to nature. You will find yourself listening to your heart and letting it lead you. Sometimes you might feel as if it has lead you astray, but upon reflection, you will find your heart knew exactly where it was leading you. Increased intuition comes to the forefront and you allow it to guide you. You become aware of your Essence, and understand we are all one. Compassion and love become gifts you generously present to all living things without even thinking of human labels such as class, religion, age, color, race, sex, or any distinction. You begin to see the world, and all that is in it, is a part of you, and treat it differently.

An increased healing of yourself, your soul, and others is experienced through creative expression. You might find you are expressing yourself through song, dance, gardening, art, speaking, coaching, writing, or anything that expresses who you are within your heart. You discover healing gifts and talents that you either didn't realize were there, or you have finally stepped out of your comfort zone and learn to express them. You gain a new perspective on life, the afterlife, the Universe, science, and spirituality. You crave information by any means possible and you absorb everything you can find. You ask the important questions and you are open to the flood of information. You are consumed with a desire to share all that you know to help others along the way.

You find yourself focusing on the present, on the truly simple things, the here and the now, and a Higher Power. You calm down and enjoy life, and understand you are on a path - a mission - which is greater than anything you had previously imagined. Everything you experience is done so through heightened senses. Spiritual awakening is the hunger to be your authentic self – your pure spirit.[1] It is the feeling within you that sends your hairs standing on end when you feel everything is as it should be; the innate feeling that the direction you are headed in is the right one. It is the electricity that comes from feeling the alignment of your character and your personality with your soul and the Universe – the creation of a clear and uninterrupted pathway between your spirit and the Divine.

---

[1] Jesus said, "If you do not bring forth what is within you, what you do not bring forth will destroy you." Didymos Judas Thomas, The Gospel of Thomas, Gnostic Gospels

We are entering the Age of Aquarius, a time for spiritual evolution, enlightenment, and ascension. We are becoming more aware, we understand the light from which we came and to which we are returning. As we find ourselves awakening, we meet more and more souls awakening as well. We seek each other out through vibrational energy and frequencies, and assist each other along our spiritual ascension.

We are connected to one another, all of us with no exclusions. We breathe each other's expended breath; our energies dance together and intermingle. We pass these energies around like an invisible pipe - all taking a drag yet never realizing the amount of smoke we are allowing into our being by doing so. The smoke (negative and positive energy) filters down into our core and produces our emotions and feelings. Positive energy can give us strength, while negative will erode our spirit. Therefore when we are not careful, or in tune, it can settle in for days, weeks, years, and even a lifetime. Energy is the one constant in our Earthly life, flowing into and out of our body with every breath, during every second of our life cycle. This energy is how the Universe functions. It is how it sustains itself as well as how it creates and destroys life. Whatever we label it, whether cosmic consciousness, God, the Universe, or Divine, energy is pure and is essential for all life as well as our soul.

The soul rides upon the motion of energy, accomplishing missions and even getting lost now and then along the journey when the mind and soul struggle over control of the body. Whatever Higher Power you hold within your heart, you know that this energy is everywhere. It's in the stillness and in the chaos. It's in the deer leaping through the grove, the bark on the tree, the water in the river, the soft petals on the flower in the park – divine energy is all encompassing. It is in all that we take in through our senses and it rides the wave – the constant flow of energy moving in and out of our own body. The breath you breathe is constantly flowing through all living things. The breath you are taking in now may have been the expended breath of a tree, or a hummingbird, or the child playing on the other side of the world.

Our soul, our spirit, is separate from our mind and body. The soul is pure consciousness – our life force. The soul lives on independently from the mind and body – even as the body dies. The body simply gives the soul a place to settle into while it is here doing its own work. Picture yourself staying at a hotel while you are out of town - except it's for a lifetime. It's not your permanent dwelling, but you will make the best of the accommodations while you are in this place. Once you make your reservation, you are there for the duration.

6

The place may or may not be comfortable. You might have wonderful neighbors around you, and you might not. The point is this place – this body – is what your soul picked for itself to for this part of its journey.

When we arrive at this place, we unpack our bags and set out on a course of learning and soul growth. Although we are in a very large class together and have the same goal of divine development, we each have a different set of lessons to learn and a different series of tests to take. Over time our souls seek out those they have traveled with before in previous journeys. If we are lucky, we come to recognize these old friends and our souls now have genuine comfort and company along their path.

These old energies are nothing at all like the majority of the energies we are surrounded with. Imagine a time when you were in school and you compared your class schedule with those of your friends. It was exciting to know you would be in the same lecture with your best friend, but most times you were in a class with people you had never met, or didn't know very well at all.

While we are always wrapped in the energy of all others, these energies are all on different frequencies. The energies we travel through time and space with are on the same vibrational level, which is why we feel overwhelming connection with some people while others are just in the room.

Our souls are constantly weaving through the tapestry of life, always striving to be divine – it is their one and only purpose. To reach that purpose, they are sent to a place where they can untangle the knots and really learn what it is they need to accomplish. The human experience will afford the soul an opportunity to feel with the body and process with the mind - thus infusing a lasting imprint upon its threads. The soul will understand pleasure and pain through the human senses, and be able to store that knowledge within itself – and carry it through space, time, and dimensions. Woven within the very fabric of the soul are all the lifetimes and lessons we've experienced. We don't always draw on this knowledge (which would make this lifetime a bit easier). I'm not sure why this is but maybe drawing upon old knowledge is considered cutting corners; maybe we are not supposed to be able to remember or view those old lessons.

When our soul arrives, we have a known mission. The same goes for those other souls that we surround ourselves with. Our visit may serve a two-fold purpose: to learn and to teach. Not all souls are here to teach us something. We might be here to help them. It may be that we surround ourselves with some people simply for the souls they themselves are connected to. We also might just be residing at the same place in this time for no other purpose except for we just happen to be occupying the same space.

Some are older souls than our own, some are younger. For this reason we live our Earthly lives with people who will never understand the concept of soul as well as those who understand it fully. We might form ties to people who have ulterior motives and live merely a material existence, those who may be consumed with the Earthly body, the ones who have not awakened yet - or are spiritually young. We might bond on some level for fun or beauty, or convenience. Even though these bonds might last a long time, they never nourish the soul in the way it needs to be nourished. It is impossible as these souls are not traveling on the same frequency. For this reason, we are constantly scanning the waves of energy for those on our own vibrational energy level. If we are lucky we will happen across other souls whom we've traveled with before and re-establish the deep connections within that higher soul level. This is why we have those uncanny feelings as if we've known this person forever, or an immediate, deep friendship develops. In them, we find home. Home in the sense of where our soul resides; that place where it is unimaginable to be without the energy they radiate; a solid state of comfort.

There's quite a big difference in the relationships we have with people we consider friends, and those we know to be of a higher connection of soul. With good friends we feel a very strong bond, but until you've had the experience of reuniting with a true soul connection, one can never understand the deep level of higher love exchanged between the energies of the two. Putting this into an Earthly example, I could cite the movie Wizard of Oz. Here you are in life, living happy and joyous with friends and family, and then all of a sudden you meet someone and your world suddenly turns from beautiful black and white to Technicolor. Although your world in black and white is satisfying and comforting, now you suddenly see that same exact world in vibrant color - flooding every single sense of your body. With a new light being shed upon your world you are able to find amazement and wonder in each and every facet of life. Your body blossoms open, your conscious unfolds to receive more of these waves of light and energy. You might find yourself with sudden bursts of creative energy around these rekindled connections.

2.

Meet the Chorus of Souls

All soul energies are connected on some level, we all interlace. In constant motion, souls are entering and exiting the different realms including Earth for the purpose of completing the next leg of their Divine journey. As the chorus of a song is always repeated several times over, so is the incarnation process of the soul.

Kindred spirits are connections that feel very warm and fuzzy, comfortable and heart-warming. Usually we find a kindred spirit in a soul that is at or near our own soul age with a vibrational energy very near to our own. Kindred spirits connect more on an energy level rather than on a higher level, but are very comforting to the soul just the same.

There are a few levels of higher connection between souls. Many times over in our Earthly life we experience the bonds between souls – those we travel together with in lifetimes. All of these levels of connection are beautiful and special. Soul connections know no boundaries in terms of gender. These connections can be established between men and women, between women, and between men. Gender is a human term, not a spiritual condition. These connections cannot be looked at in terms of relationships here on Earth. Over the span of lifetimes within a soul, we establish many connections and travel in the same circles with each other. It is not at all comparable to the Earthly notion of picking a partner and remaining with them.

There are also different levels of soul connection. We don't always travel with the same souls, but some we travel with more frequently. In some lifetimes these connections in Earthly bodies are in different types of Earthly relationships. Sometimes we are lovers; sometimes friends; sometimes family; sometimes complete strangers. Our soul energy stores the imprints we've made throughout lifetimes, and this is the reason we might meet someone and feel an instant draw to them. It's not a draw of sexual energy, but a draw of soul energy. A true soul connection runs so deeply that Earthly words cannot describe the bond. We tend to feel it with heightened senses, or as if the path ahead of us is illuminated.

When we reestablish these connections in a new lifetime, we might feel as if we've known them our whole life, but we can't put our finger on why we feel this way. It's a draw, a pull toward one another.

Twin Souls

When new souls are born from the Divine Source, the energy of that soul is split into two - forming two souls that share a powerful energy source, yet are independent souls on their own. They are polar opposites of their spiritual counterparts; the Yin and the Yang: one with female tendencies and the other with male tendencies. (Not in terms of gender but in terms of principal). But they also contain parts of the other. Once reunited after all their own soul work is done, they will join back again into one energy.

We call these Twin Souls (or Twin Flames). They incarnate separately gathering lessons and experiences over and over again, lifetime after lifetime. The vibrational level of these souls is the same. Generally they don't incarnate together very often, but due to the big shift in consciousness lately, they are finding each other sooner. Unless their individual souls have evolved (how they've learned and dealt with their lessons in Earthly life) the meeting may be difficult and they may separate once again, and attempt it later. This is the most intense of soul connections and it is the strongest attraction of spirit, therefore, if when they meet they are not at the same place - soulfully - it will be a painful and oftentimes difficult experience. All their individual healing and emotional baggage must be dealt with and finished before these two can meet in a lifetime without pain. Each must be in balance and aligned with their tendencies, their energy, their Yin or Yang - in order to be rejoined fully and completely with their twin, and only at that point will they be whole in the spiritual sense.

Twin Souls are always connected, even when one has not incarnated and is still in a higher realm and the other is on, for instance, the Earthly plane. The love between twin souls is an unconditional, sacred love of the highest spiritual bond. It is not romantic love as we experience in a human or an Earthly sense, it is much deeper than that. Think of it on a cosmic level. When the two become one again, they form a single consciousness. Their love is pure, it is eternal, and it is magnetic. It is divine.

When Twin Souls connect on Earth it can be very difficult. What makes one off kilter, or off center, usually is also seen in the other twin. One is working on theirs from the Yin perspective and the other from their Yang perspective. Each of them holds a piece of what the other needs for healing the wounds of the other, and what they need for the growth of each other's soul. They may find themselves with incredible bursts of creativity during their time together. They are generally always in sync no matter if they are in the same dimension or not. However, should they meet in the physical world, the energy would be very intense and wonderfully explosive; immediately a soul connection would be realized, provided they are both at the same level to understand this and be aware of this. Again, I am not talking about lovers, I am talking about cosmic love – love in a pure, authentic, spiritual form. Although if they did meet in the physical world, it would be a completely intense dynamic, not like the majority of what is felt through human relationships. As with other soul connections and relationships, a reunion of such souls does not mean you will spend your Earthly existence with them, it merely means you are here at this time together to grow spiritually. Soul inspired love, soul family and soul mates all help us to heal ourselves and heal each other so that we can spread that love to humanity and the major shift in consciousness that is taking place can further develop and progress.

Although a rare occurrence for both halves of the twin soul to be Earthbound together at the same time, it does happen. It can be difficult because chances are they are each in their own human relationships. This is where pain and confusion comes in. The ease of which this can be dealt with depends upon the age and place the soul is in here on Earth. It is important to keep in mind that Earthly, or human, relationships serve a purpose in the lessons and healing of the soul and need to be maintained in order for that soul to progress. Not all twin souls that unite in a given lifetime will do so romantically, nor should they. Depending upon how awake the part of their soul is that has incarnated at the time – will determine if it is even possible for that soul to recognize their twin. Sometimes one knows and the other can't fathom the concept. In this case the one who is more awake must practice patience. Sometimes neither is ready within their soul journey. Sometimes both are ready spiritually for the connection in whatever form presents itself. More often than not, even when twin souls incarnate at the same time, they (whether one or both) remain unconscious of the connection until such time as their personality is aligned with their soul rather than the ego, and they are healed from the wounds they have accumulated in life and ready spiritually to accept that connection.

Soul Family

The souls we travel with more frequently are our soul family. When you are on the Earthly plane and a member of your soul family seeks you out, it is quite an amazing and profound meeting of energies. These are our Beloveds. It is a connection centered in the heart. Soul family is one of highest connections you can have spiritually. Soul brothers, sisters, parents, etc. Soul family members travel with each other and make the choice to do so. They incarnate together, but they don't necessarily end up together in the sense of the Earthly family unit. They know what lessons you have to learn, and you know what lessons they have to learn. Everyone can work on their karma by supporting each other as a soul family. You love each other so deeply at the soul level that you choose to filter into each other lives (your paths cross,) to assist each other in learning the things you have to learn individually. Just as it is here on Earth, you might prefer to hang out with or gravitate toward certain people in your life, so the same goes for souls in your soul family.

How do you know when you've met a soul from your soul family? There is an instant draw, pull, or uncanny attraction that is unexplainable and deeper than anything you can imagine. It is that feeling like you've known someone your entire life although you have just met for the first time. The best way I can describe it is that there is a feeling of home. An unexplainable feeling of love is radiated, an authentic love. It is a very special connection that you will come to hold precious, although you might not understand it fully at first.

The fact that you are in an Earthly body with an Earthly mind might make things complicated. Unless you are completely advanced spiritually, the ties experienced, the bond, the connection - are going to be interpreted with the mind and the body first. You will unavoidably put this relationship into the context of Earthly terms, and give it an Earthly label. You might feel the draw as a parent, lover, child, or whatever you were to each other in a former lifetime. These connections run so incredibly deep that there are no definitions for them.

Much of the confusion may lie in the fact that you do have imprints of your past connection upon your soul. You will pick up on these somewhat in the current life as your energies connect with one another. The fact that you traveled in past lifetimes as lovers, family or whatever your past Earthly relationship was, will be very confusing and difficult to set aside in this lifetime. The key is to try your hardest to put down the Earthly labels and understand that it is just an incredibly deep love, on a very high and spiritual level. By love I don't mean in the physical sense, but in terms of divine love.

Soul family members reuniting will have an instant, unexplainable bond that develops. You think alike, have the same interests, and are shoved together it seems by some unknown force. You share the same ideas and understand what each other are thinking about, and talking about, with little to no effort. Your energy and their energy connect fast and furious and you experience a feeling of "coming home," of being content, happy, and at ease – within your core. You are very aware of the connection you have and at first you cannot explain it. Sometimes, much like the connective energy of twin babies, soul energy can be so strong that pain or joy can be sensed without direct communication.

We connect at odd times in our lives and seemingly out of the blue. Sometimes they pop into our lives for a short while, and sometimes they are in our lives for a long time. This can explain why some people make a profound impact on us even though we didn't know them long, and others can seemingly come into our lives randomly as strangers and remain with us as good friends until we die. Usually, soul family will welcome each other, love and cherish each other – expanding their journey on a much higher level than on an Earthly dimension.

Depending where you are spiritually in your current lifetime, you may or may not be able to handle these Beloveds entering your life. You may not even see them on the deeper spiritual level; you may embrace them right away; you may need to take a while to understand it and process it.

Souls incarnate together to help one another progress in each other's journeys. You understand what lessons the other needs to learn. Therefore, when you meet in a lifetime you are there to aid each other's soul progression through earthly relationship. The connection is so interwoven, so strong, that through all the confusion you will find the ability to free your soul of unresolved matters that might be inhibiting your journey at the present time. Beloveds push each other's buttons on a higher level, causing them to look deep and understand what issues they need to deal with. Issues you are dragging with you that you need to let go of; issues that require the energy of a Beloved to help you to overcome and advance in your ascension of spirit.

Once you are able to strip away the human description of the connection, and understand that it is a connection seated in another dimension, it will be much easier to accept the love and light of each other and continue the progression of soul evolution. There might be times when you revert to a mortal thought or feeling, once again trying to attach an earthly emotion or label upon the connection. That is only natural considering you are living a very human existence after all, and considering the intermingling your energies have experienced over lifetimes of travel together, and the ego based relationships you have experienced in past connections, it makes perfect sense for these powerful feelings to crop back up once in a while. It is a matter of separating that which you know to be an earthly sensation from that which you know is a spiritual connection.

Meeting a member of your soul family can be a very painful experience at times because they force you to put aside Earthly expression on one hand, while forcing you to take a long hard look at yourself on the other hand. They help you to illuminate your flaws and the things you fear by directing you inward to face them. Soul family members are an incredibly powerful ally and aid in the evolution of your soul.

When you connect with members of your soul family a new world opens up to you. A place where all there is – is divine love. Putting aside earthly description you will be able to recreate that feeling here on Earth and make your stay more enjoyable. It is a place where you are open to receive love and to give love (authentically and unconditionally) just as it is on that higher plane of the Divine. Beloveds also help us to open up the door so that more of these connections can enter our earthly experience. They may remain until our soul is seated in contentment and its current journey is eased and able to continue on its path surrounded by love and light. Once you open up the lines of energy that you possess and let them unfold, you will attract more love and light, more authentic connections, and you will become able to see, and to expand, your authentic self.

Soul Mates

We often hear the term soul mates. Soul mates are strong connections similar to our soul family. I wish the word "mate" weren't attached to this term because it is generally brings up images of the Earthly "mate" and that isn't at all what it means. A soul mate is not someone that is your one and only true love for all eternity, forever and ever, amen. Sometimes in an Earthly life you might be married to this person, but more often than not that is not the case.

Soul mates most often support each other, love each other unconditionally and are here to add to or enrich each other's existence in this lifetime. Again, we are not at all referring to the romantic love as we know it be on Earth, but a cosmic love, a pure and spiritual love. It is a love that travels time, space, and dimensions. Having a soul mate doesn't mean they will be in our life for all time, nor does it mean the two will get married and live happily ever after. You will have more than one soul mate and you might find these relationships in the form of lovers, friends, family, co-workers or neighbors. You will also come to realize that these souls with whom you travel don't incarnate in the same forms of relationship all the time. Sometimes you might be lovers, sometimes friends, sometimes family. You may be coworkers or internet friends. Sometimes soul mates may even be your enemies, abusers, or someone who does harm to you. It's all about in the lessons we need to learn, the things we need to work on for our soul, and these connections are here to help us do this. Soul mates are not forever and they do not always make us feel good.

During our stint on Earth, we develop personalities and traits. These come as a result of what we are taught, what we learn and what we came here with. They are a result of our environment, our friends, our family, and our experiences. We have to develop a way to navigate our spirit through and around these personalities and traits as our soul journeys in this lifetime. A soul connection will help you to clear your path, looking at where you have been and where you are going. They will give you the strength to make adjustments and discard unhealthy ego based feelings attached to your being. They will help you to align your earthly traits and personality with your soul energy. When that happens and a direct path is cleared between the two planes, you have the clarity you need to move forward. You don't need a soul connection to be able to do this, but it certainly is a welcomed embrace that flows from the Divine.

A soul is energy. It is your divine light. It is origin of your intuition. A soul, once divinely born, must set out on a journey to become part of its Source. In order to do this, the soul is born into a tangible form, like a human body for instance, in order to experience learning by using tools available in that body, such as the senses. The soul's goal is to be in harmony, to love and be loved unconditionally, to be compassionate, to free itself from earthly illusion, and to hold all life in the highest regard. These goals, once mastered, will ascend the soul back to the Source. We learn from The Bhagavad Gita[2], "*The one who discerns: what deserves attention and what does not, what ought to be done and what ought not to be, what ought to be bewared of and what ought not to be, what is slavery and what is freedom — the one who can differentiate this has a developed consciousness and lives in sattva.*[3]"

When we are born we develop personalities and traits. They come from our parents, our surroundings, our friends, and everyone we are touched by in our lifetime. Our body and our mind are affected by these personalities and traits, as well as by our character, our

---

[2] The Bhagavad Gita – Song of God – 18: 30.
[3] Sattva: Hindu, meaning purity, lightness, balanced

24

habits (good or bad) and how we experience and interpret life. We are multi-sensory and relate everything in terms of our Earthly senses. At some point in our life on Earth we develop another sense – the sense that there is something more. I like to call it the sense of home.

The sense of home is the innate realization that there is much more to life than our Earthly existence. Something bigger, unexplainable, somewhere we know we have come from before we were born, and somewhere we know we will return to when we die. The sense of home is about as important as all the other Earthly senses combined and the one that takes the most time to develop. The key to experiencing, or finding, our sense of home is to align ourselves with our own soul. To do this we need to understand ourselves and our way of thinking. When we delve into our inner self, we will understand how our senses have helped form our personality and made us who we are in this Earthly body and mind. We can work on understanding the how and the whys of the way we feel about people, things, situations; we can work on understanding how to let go of the feelings that do not serve our soul; we can correct the habits that force our souls to be misaligned and slowly push us off our soul's path.

The goal is to align our character with our soul – to clear a path in the Universe between your soul and home.

25

Everyone feels the result of this from time to time. It is the feeling that everything is going right in your life; it is a happiness that resonates throughout your body and mind; it is the feeling that you are on the right path. The pathway opens for you as you rid yourself from negative energy in your life. It's the feeling you get when you finally break a bad habit. It's also the experience of doing something good for another soul, or opening yourself up to something new that really feels right in your heart of hearts.

All religions teach the importance of clearing a path between the soul and home – it's being the best that you can be. It a matter of understanding the need to do this and to incorporate it into your earthly life, because when the time does come for you to go home, you will be taking some of this earthly stuff – this personality, this character - with you because it is so strong it leaves an imprint upon your soul.

When you return home you will watch the ripple effect of your life now gone. You will see how the words and actions you let out into the Universe has affected those who were around you. How it infused into their own personalities and life's lessons, and you will be amazed on how far the ripples reach. You will see how ripples from others affected you and how you in turn affected the souls of others. Each of us is important and we each have some purpose to fulfill here on Earth. Our souls are in training; our souls are here to learn – to grow and mature. Earth is but a boot camp for the soul. Through the senses and our many lives here, our soul accomplishes its mission. Many lifetimes make a soul divine, and each time we are reborn we have one more opportunity to work on our divinity.

"Mans forgetfulness of his divine resources (the result of his misuse of free will) is the root cause of all other forms of suffering."[4]
Paramahansa Yogananda

---

[4] *The Autobiography of a Yogi* by Paramahansa Yogananda, Originally Published 1946

3.

Earth U

What if you were told you were going to be sent somewhere? This place, you are told, will have a lot of obstacles; it will present you with both pleasant and difficult situations. You are told it will be your task to navigate through this place, these situations, using grace, love, compassion, and patience.

The manner in which you weave yourself through this present place – how you meet your challenges and most importantly what you learn from the inhabitants and tribulations of this place – will determine the next place you will visit. It will play a big factor on what you will face in the next place – the people, situations, circumstances, and its level of difficulty. The foundation of the next place you visit will be rooted in what you accomplished (or didn't accomplish) in the present place.

What if you were told that you had in your possession certain tools to use in order to maintain strength of mind and aid in a more successful completion of your goals in this place? Tools that you already have within you – you cannot physically see them but are within you.

What if you were told you will not be alone in this place – there will be people and animals and many living examples there to help you to meet your goals. You, in turn, might help them meet theirs. You would be sharing the space with many others who have the same goal but have an entirely different set of circumstances and obstacles to navigate through. Even the ones who appear to sabotage your goals are there to help you through strength from your reactions. Some will be there for the duration of stay in this place while others will pop in for a short period.

Welcome to Earth University. Tuition is free. Attendance is mandatory. Failure is not an option, but some courses may need to be repeated.

When you came here your soul already knew what its purpose would be this time around. It arrived with the clear understanding of what it needed in order to correct or perfect itself. From the family you chose (whether the natural born or adopted) – you knew ahead of time where you would be and the environment you would live in. Your soul selected this life ahead of time so the work it needed to complete would be completed within a favorable environment for its lessons.

When you completely understand that it was your soul that selected your life, you can begin to move forward and begin the process of healing the spirit and reinforcing the positive parts. Your soul is your authentic self. It's the real you. It is who you are when you are at your finest; when you are experiencing the alignment with home, with God, the Universe, or with a Higher Power. All life is, is about alignment. Think about it, when you are feeling positive you are feeling good mentally and physically you do good things for people and you feel happiness inside yourself deep down. You are healthier. When you are in alignment (between your soul and home) you are at your most powerful self. You are in balance. Life seems to go a bit smoother, you see little things you might have otherwise not paid attention to. You learn to find gratitude and appreciation in everything. Hard times might be reflected upon as lessons; you will see the positive in the bad circumstances and you will begin to understand how you can let go of the negative more freely and more often.

Every time you feel unbalanced, unhealthy, unhappy, or out of whack – chances are you have fallen out of alignment. Your health and well-being are directly related to your soul alignment. If you are not serving your soul with what you are doing or thinking, you are out of sorts – there is not a clear path between your soul and the

31

Divine. Life becomes a thick foggy night with you trudging through, squinting in the dark, trying to make your way. It's hard to breathe and the air seems to hang about you. Your health may suffer or you may become ill, depressed, or make bad choices.

In a lifetime you will go through bouts of alignment as well as misalignment. It's not as if once you are aligned you are going to remain that way for your whole life. That's not the way it works – not for the majority of humanity, anyhow. They key idea is to be able to ride out your own storms with the knowledge that you alone have the power within yourself to break through, break free, and give yourself a break. Understand whatever it is that is hindering your soul's journey, whatever it is that is making you feel down, negative, or just not right – can be overcome by using the gifts that you arrived here with.

Your soul holds these cherished gifts for you and all you have to do is to allow yourself to use them. These gifts are the art of letting go (by this I mean letting go of hurt, pain, emotions – not necessarily people although once in a while that too is necessary), the art of inner peace and personal space, and the all the beautiful, divine tools contained within the seed of the soul.

4.

Sacred Seeds

You came here possessing a seed: a seed of sacred knowledge. One which contains everything you will need in your lifetime as your soul journeys. As children we nourish the seed by being open and honest, inquisitive and pure, and we have the innate ability to express unconditional love – while absorbing our world as it is and finding the joy, wonder and enjoyment in each moment. Over the formative years and as we age, the seed becomes neglected. As our personalities and our character develop, the way we look at the world becomes different and skewed by our perceptions of life. We've learned about race, religion, gender, sexuality, lifestyles, and class. Opinions, for good or bad, have formed through our family, friends, and environment. We no longer allow our mind to freely love and accept as we had done as a child – stipulations are attached to everything we think and feel.

Our seed lays dormant waiting for us to grow up and rediscover our purpose. It waits patiently for us to find our inner child and begin once again to cultivate a life of compassion, love, and authenticity. Whether it is a case of getting to your breaking point or feeling like something has got to give; maybe you're searching for something bigger than yourself or you just have many more questions than answers – this is the point where a personal journey begins. This is when you dig deep for that seed and begin to unlock the wonder it holds for personal growth.

At this point you must separate all the learned behavior from that which you know to be sacred knowledge. For instance, you might realize that loving all religions even though they are not in line with your own beliefs is the divine way. This creates respect and love and strengthens your character. As you go about on your soul journey you will nurture this Sacred Seed and through tending it will foster tolerance, unconditional love, compassion, gratitude, and forgiveness. All of these qualities will help you overcome the negative things you have experienced in life. Through them you will learn that even though you cannot stop yourself from experiencing negative things, you have the tools within you to get through these things quickly and without dwelling on them.

You will come to understand with your whole heart that these negative things do not define you. It's simply a matter of how you deal with circumstances, and what you do with that energy, that moves you forward or, holds you back.

Chorus of Souls

5.

Create a Healthy Spiritual Practice

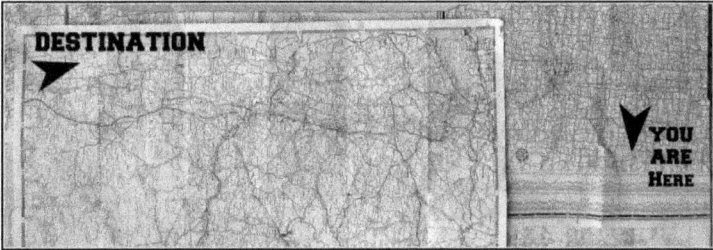

We are all on different paths to the same place. It is the place we know to be our Divine Home. Picture a map spread out before you on a long table. We are all on one end of the map and we all have to get to the other end of the map. Picture religion, no religion, or the equivalent of religion is your mode of transportation. Now, some of us might take a train; other may fly. A few might walk; some may ride a bike, a horse, or an elephant. If we drive a car it could be an old clunker, a shiny sports car, or anything in between. There are infinite routes (ways of living) that can be set out upon – some are more direct and some meander all over the place. The terrain could be hilly or smooth, crooked or straight; the climate could be cold or hot; the food source could be abundant or scarce. Whichever method we start out with might change at some point along the way. There is nothing about this journey that is mandatory. It doesn't matter how you arrive at the destination, nor the amount of time it shall take you to arrive. The point is, we are all here, we will all be going back home, and the circumstances along the way really don't matter as long as we learn from them.

Cultivating one's spiritual practice requires daily commitment and patience. You constantly reinforce your spirit through practicing the fine arts of love, compassion, grace, patience, and being conscious about every single thing around you.

There are some wonderful travel guides we have available to us though, for our journey! Things that don't cost a dime and are readily available anytime we need them. When we make use of these guides, our journey is a more calm, balanced, and less stressful. They will put meaning in the time we are here, and benefit us greatly. Let's explore these guides.

Being Present

If you put a bucket into a stream and scoop up a heap of rock, sand, and water – this is like the mind. Looking into the bucket, we see a muddy, cloudy mess. It takes a few minutes of letting the bucket sit still (without touching it) so that the contents settle. The rocks will fall to the bottom of the bucket, and as the sand separates from the water it settles beneath the rock allowing the water to slowly become clear.

All of the things that were mixed with the water when you first scooped it up – remain in the bucket. All that swirled randomly around moments ago is now quiet and settled. Every space of the bucket is filled, but there is order and stillness so that each item can be clearly identified. The same holds true for the mind. If you want to quiet the mind, you must give yourself time to rest and settle.

So you might be thinking, "Good analogy but how do you actually do this?" First you need to be committed to practicing it. You must have patience. When you are present it means you are focused on what you are doing at the moment. You're not doing three things at one time, but you are turning your attention to one thing. This means when you are eating – you are just eating; when you are at your kid's ballgame – you are paying attention to the game, to your child. You are not on your cell or multi-tasking.

Take time out each and every day just for yourself. Use this time to relax, meditate, pray, have a cup of coffee in silence, or whatever you like, as long as it involves you and only you. If you've never allowed yourself to do this before, start slow with five or ten minutes and work your way up to an hour or so. Sit outside and enjoy the sights

39

and sounds of nature; take a walk and let your surroundings fill your senses; concentrate on the feel and sound of your breath as you sit in stillness and quiet. Don't think of anything except for what your senses are picking up at the moment. Nature is essential to your soul; nature is essential to your health.

When you are having a conversation with someone, listen to what the other person is saying. Don't be distracted by thinking of what you are going to say next, or what you want to make for dinner that evening. Do not answer text messages or phone calls. Focus solely on the conversation.

Stop worrying. Every time you see yourself thinking about something in the future, stop it! Bring yourself back to the present moment and remain there. If you are studying for a test, don't worry about the test – when you do you have just spent less time studying for it. If you are writing a speech – don't worry about how nervous you will be – when you do this you will have less time to write a quality speech. Surrender your fantasy of the outcome, do your best, and accept whatever happens. Taking the time to remain in the moment enhances whatever you are doing in that space.

"A wandering mind is human nature.
Every time your thoughts get off subject, simply return to the present.
Don't try to not think about the thought, because the more you try
not to think of it, the more you are thinking of it!
Instead, just dismiss it and get back to the subject of your focus.
Immerse yourself in things that normally you wouldn't pay attention
to. Be the conductor of your own orchestra, directing your senses to
savor every aspect of your immersion."[5]

---

[5] Excerpt from *Booyah! Spirit: 52 Ingredients for a Healthy Soul. Suffering is Optional* by Sheila M. Burke

Forgive

Definition[6]:

To stop feeling angry or resentful towards someone for an offence, flaw, or mistake. To no longer feel angry about or wish to punish.

Notice the definition says nothing whatsoever about being content with the things that happened to you, or the things said about you. Forgiveness is not about being a doormat and letting the other person walk all over you. To forgive is to let go and heal your own spirit.

Forgiveness comes when you understand people are doing the best that they can – with the tools they have unlocked from within. Sometimes they have not located the proper tools yet, so they are doing the best they can with what they understand.

By not forgiving, you place yourself into the perpetual cycle of reliving and retelling the same stories over and over again. Reliving the pain and anger, harboring resentment, judgment, and all those negative feelings you retain when you feel you have been wronged. You are stuck. This negative energy affects you in your everyday life, in your thoughts, in your sleep, in your

---

[6] Oxford Dictionary

daydreams. It walks with you everywhere you go. It starts to fiddle with you on a cellular level, your cells vibrate slower, causing upset and illness. It breaks you down and affects your spirit.

Carrying the burden of resentment or regret is not unlike running a 5K while draped in a twice insulated, ankle length coat. There is absolutely no need to do this, and upon removing the burden, you realize how much lighter you feel.

We carry resentment because someone has made us feel as if we didn't measure up to their expectations about us. Nasty words or actions come from a place of pain and suffering, and how we respond to them also comes from a place of pain and suffering. You cannot make the past better. It is over and done with. What happened happened, and the only way to grow is to look ahead, and move forward.

Tips on Forgiving

Keep in mind we are all on different paths and in different places in our spiritual growth. Remind yourself how you would like to be treated, if the roles were reversed, or if it were you who was not being forgiven.

Ask yourself, when you die will you say, "I wish I had remained angry longer," or "I wish I wasted more time being resentful?"

Try to picture this person as a child and remember somewhere inside they are still that child – a child that will make mistakes.

Ask yourself, "If I remove this persons offending behavior, would I still love them for who they are in my life?"

When you think of their offending behavior, replace that thought with a thought of love and compassion.

Remember that whatever they said or did, it was about them, and not about you. They are responsible for their own words and actions.

Remember how you felt the last time you were forgiven. Keep in mind everyone is broken at some point in their life. It is not your job to fix them, but it is your job to fix you. Forgiving *them* heals *you*.

How to Forgive

Acknowledge your emotion

Find a friend, if you need to, that you can trust, that is able to be quiet and listen to your pain as you express your feelings. You do not want to unburden your emotions to someone who is going to reinforce your reason for having not forgiven the other person. You need to talk with someone who is able to listen and let you unburden. The objective is not to re-hash or re-live by retelling your story over and over as if you are seeking approval – the goal is to get it out, once and for all, and begin using the tips on forgiving.

Write down your feelings, how you feel the emotion, where you feel the emotion, what it is doing to you mentally and physically. Cry if you need too, scream if you have to. Write a letter to this person detailing how you feel and why. It will be the letter you write, but never send because you are confronting them only through confronting the experience within you. As go through the steps of forgiving, you will burn this letter – and as the smoke ascends you will literally be able to visualize letting go of the burden. Experience the emotions.

Take a breather and calm down.

Ideally, what would you like to happen to this emotion? Where would you like it to go, and what would you be comfortable replacing it with?

Make a plan

Ask yourself how you can make it happen. What simple steps can you take to rid yourself of your feelings towards this person? Step back and take a breather – allowing some distance between the two of you and some time to practice your tips on forgiveness.

Understand it may all revisit you.

While it sounds great, this is a learning process. It takes a lot work, a lot of patience, and commitment. Being unable to forgive is much like having an addiction. It takes time and effort to rid yourself from it.

Be Grateful

Being grateful is extremely important to the health of your soul. When we are grateful for what we have, we find that we no longer focus on what we feel is missing or what we think we are lacking. Finding gratitude in what we already have encourages a positive attitude, positive energy, and love of life. Being grateful for all that you have right now helps you to connect with yourself and will keep you in the present moment.

No matter what your situation is, if you are alive, you have something to be thankful for in your life. Being grateful fosters a healthy well-being. We are no longer putting our energy into what we lack; instead we are feeling good about what we do have. When you are no longer longing for something, we are better able to appreciate all that we do have. Our mood lightens, we smile more, and we are far less stressed. Gratitude also strengthens our relationships, and helps us to be more forgiving. We find joy inside things that we might not have seen before. Being grateful calms us down, and when we are calm we experience a good vibration within our cells, our blood pressure lowers, and we tend to take better care of ourselves.

Being grateful is not only about material things, and is not confined to the good things that we have or that happen to us. Learning to be grateful is almost like an art.

We have to ponder, we have to reach deep sometimes, to find the brighter side of something and be thankful for it. A car accident where no one was seriously injured is a blessing, something to find gratitude in. When you're upset because a law states that you can no longer smoke in your workplace, you realize this is the perfect opportunity to quit smoking. Your children's school events have filled your calendar for the next two weeks – find gratitude in spending quality time enjoying your children.

People who are awakening will find gratitude in the ordinary, the mundane, the difficult, the joyful, the sad, the hurt, the amazing, the weird, the absurd, the tragic, the enjoyable, and the mess. They will find appreciation everywhere and it will become, for them, something extraordinary. It's found at the point where you can take a feeling or situation and really look inside of it – beyond the first impression, behind the surface.

Look deeper when you find something to be grateful for. It's easy to say you are grateful for the sunset, but why are you grateful? How does it make you feel? What do you experience? Maybe you feel grateful for the day cooling down, how the colors warm you, or because it relaxes your mind. Experience your gratitude on the core, or spiritual level. You will learn to find beauty, love, and appreciation for all that you encounter in life. You will come to the understanding that we are all one, we are all connected, and you will nourish your soul on a deep level. Gratitude for everything, including that which may seem insignificant, creates a peaceful environment for yourself while sending ripples of peace out into the world around you.

Be grateful out loud! When you are thankful for something, express yourself. Imagine the trend we could start by simply expressing how grateful we are for the little things in our day to another soul. They will start looking for the things that they too are thankful for, and they will take that experience with them as they go about their day – continuing the wave of gratitude.

Every day write down a few things in which you are grateful for, or keep a gratitude journal. Encourage your children to practice gratitude in the same way; young children can draw pictures about what they are thankful for. Gratitude journals are wonderful for children; they make great gifts for all ages. Visit your local craft store and create a beautiful journal for yourself or someone you love. A beautiful place dedicated to recording your thoughts is very helpful in the follow through of daily gratitude.

Use the words "thank you" and "I appreciate you" often. Say them with your authentic self, from the heart. By understanding how grateful you are, you are transforming your energy and connecting with Source.

You are announcing your appreciation for all that you have been given, and when that happens you will attract more goodness and happiness into your life.

Gratefulness fosters compassion and empathy. You will notice when you become grateful for all that you have, you feel the need to show kindness and love to others. You may realize that for all the complaining you do because your wardrobe is not up-to-date, there are many out there who do not have a coat to wear in the middle of winter. You become grateful for the clothes you do have now, and you are compelled to donate what you cannot use to a shelter. Once you stop complaining about your job, it may suddenly become apparent that many others are out of work and having trouble putting food on the table. You are thankful for being able to provide even if it is a struggle, and you find compassion to donate to a food bank or volunteer at a soup kitchen.

Finding gratitude is one of the easiest ways to make your heart happy and being compassionate is one of the easiest ways to make someone else's heart happy. Gratefulness should start first thing in the morning upon waking. It should be the foundation of your day. In the simple act of practicing gratefulness, we nourish the chorus of souls.

Service

By investing ourselves in others, we invest in our own soul. It is only when we give of ourselves in service to others, that we find meaning in our own life. When we are able to humble ourselves through compassion, kindness, caring, and love for others – it is at that point when we connect with Source.

Something happens on a cellular level when we give of ourselves. Our cells dance and delight in the circulation of love moving throughout our body. Positive and healthy energy is radiated from our being and is absorbed by those around us. Our soul has quenched its desire to be love and give love.

Humanity is Awakening!
How to join in:

Spread peace

Save a species

Be Inspiring

LIVE GREEN

Feed the hungry

love the earth

Take up a cause

Eat healthy

GIVE MORE. TAKE LESS

Love your Neighbor

help the animals

SAVE THE PLANET

Put your heart into something loving
and give it your all.

Embrace Your Purpose

The occupation you have may not be your life's purpose – and that's okay! I think we have to learn to distinguish between the two. While it would be amazing and wonderful to have the two enmesh, the fact is, most of us do not experience life in that way. Our occupation feeds our family and pays our bills – and while we might not always love what we do – it is how we earn our income. That doesn't mean we can confuse what we do for a living, with what we do for our lifetime. Working on your inner self does not mean you must change your occupation or find one conducive to your personal journey. Soul work can be separate from your Earthly occupation.

With that said, it is very important to do discover the things that make you happy, and to do those things. Ask yourself, "What makes me happy?" When you feel a yearning to do something – accomplish something – say something – share something – experience something – then you must pursue that yearning. Remember when we were kids? We would start playing; we would lose all track of time. We were so engrossed, so absorbed, in the things we loved to do. We lived in the present moment; there was no such thing as *time*.

As children we found freedom and love simply by immersing in ourselves in that which made us happy and

53

fed our soul. We possessed an intrinsic understanding that the soul and the natural world are not separate. We spent hours in nature whether playing in the creek, running in the woods, laughing and giggling in the snow, or twirling in the rain. Think as your childlike self would think. Find something that matters to you, something that aligns with your soul. When you fail to express yourself and nurture your purpose, the suppressed energy will manifest itself as anger, jealousy, discontent, and other negative feelings. If you can end up making a living while attending to your life's purpose, well then that is icing on the cake!

We are all creative beings. We all have passions. We all were created to share ourselves, our joys, our passions with the world. Whether it's writing, music, art, design, crafting, inventing, wood-working, helping people or animals, or the millions of wonderful things that make us who we are – *we all have something that makes our soul sing.* The problem is many people think of these as a hobby which they devote a minimal amount of time.

Pay attention to how these things make you feel when you are engaged in them. Your cells are vibrating and happy; your mind gets focused; you become calm. You are aligning your soul with your personality and clearing a direct path between them in the Universe. It feels good and right. If your passions are not your

54

occupation you must make time in your day or night to include them into your life. No excuses.

Consider your creativeness a necessary part of your day – it is no different than eating. You eat to nourish your body – you *create* to nourish your soul.

Make Good Use of Your Time

Eighty percent of our thoughts are filled with meaningless garbage. Imagine what you could do, be, and feel if that percentage was turned around. What if we flipped that number? What if the eighty percent were filled with the things that nourished the soul?

What if instead of complaining how disheveled your garden is, you went out and tended to it? What if instead of reading a tabloid on your lunch break, you read a good book? What if instead of watching television, you decided to take a walk? What if instead of watching a reality show on television, you decided to watch a nature documentary or something that actually nourished your mind? What if instead of worrying what you will wear to work or school tomorrow, you studied for a test or presentation?

What if instead of gossiping with a friend, you decided to help your child with homework, volunteer at a soup kitchen, or clean out your closets?

Make a conscious choice to utilize your time in a positive and productive manner. Take time daily to pray, meditate, be grateful, and create as all these practices will lighten and open you up to giving and receiving love. Take time for yourself every day for the same reasons. Unplug from technology and plug into your spirituality.

Develop a Daily Ritual

We've seen ritual incorporated into daily life for thousands of years. Rituals help us to stay focused and bring our mind back to a place of clarity and calm. Waking up, brushing our teeth, having a cup of coffee, reading the paper or a book, sitting outside with nature for a few minutes before you start your day – are examples of ritual just the same as going to church on Sunday or receiving communion is also a ritual. Wedding ceremonies are rituals, as are funerals. We perform rituals all the time – whether it's taking three practice swings and using our favorite lucky ball during our golf game, or taking a few deep breaths and jumping up and down a few times before running out onto the stage – we find comfort in ritual.

Rituals give us a certain confidence and draw our attention to the present moment helping us to focus on the task at hand. Rituals can also aid in the grieving process, as seen through the ways we honor our dead. The same can be said for burning rituals such as writing a letter of forgiveness that will never be sent, but instead will be burned to release the pain from your mind. As the smoke rises, the pain goes with it.

Your daily rituals set the tone for your day. Whether it's waking up thirty minutes before your children and meditating – or remaining in bed for a short time after waking for the purpose of setting a daily intention – establish your daily ritual and use it to build or maintain your spiritual tone for the day.

When the sun rises, it should be a reminder to set a good tone for the day. What do you want this day to be? Will you need strength to get through something? Will you need patience to deal with someone? Do you intend to find something wonderful everywhere you cast your eyes? What are you grateful for this day?

When the sun is setting, it should be a reminder to reflect upon your day. How did I live today? Could I have been more patient? Did I show compassion to someone? What could I have done differently in this situation, or in conveying that thought? Did I appreciate all that that this day has presented to me?

Prayer

People pray for all sorts of reasons and to all sorts of gods depending upon their religion. To cover all bases here, I'll refer to prayer as communication with one's Source. This way it encompasses all religions as well as the nontheistic.

Prayer is a way of expressing love and appreciation. It is a way in which we honor our Source. Praying doesn't mean we are begging for things, it is more about taking time throughout your day to converse with Source just as if you are having a conversation with a flesh and blood person. We pray to receive strength, express our thankfulness, and ask for guidance. We pray for ourselves and for others. What we receive from prayer might not always be what we had anticipated. Sometimes we ask for something and receive it through an obstacle. It might not become apparent until long after we've removed the obstacle. We learn through everything we are given.

Something happens in the brain when we pray. I believe it is the point where science meets Source. Many experiments have been conducted on prayer for self and prayer for others. Neural connections change within the brain during prayer and meditation. Studies, including those by famed neuroscientist Andrew Newberg, show a large decrease in parietal lobe activity which is the area of the brain that controls the way you orient to three-dimensional space. So the ability to figure out where one thing ends and another thing begins is decreased, which would indicate the feeling of being one with the Source. Activity in the frontal lobe, which is responsible for our ability to concentrate, is greatly increased.

This new field of study involving prayer or spirituality, and the brain is called Neurotheology.[7] Interestingly enough, the same results are not produced from the atheistic brain when they are asked to pray only the brain that has a belief in Source presents these results.

It is really no secret that prayer, as well as meditation, not only works, but is therapeutic. We've known this for millennia through eastern philosophies. The power of prayer can be seen and it can be measured. Maybe not up to snuff for the scientific community, just yet, and maybe it never will be. We know by the study of random number generators, that there is an increased output of energy when large groups of people focus (meditate, concentrate, pray) on the same purpose. In large groups with people all focused on the same intent or feeling we can literally feel the air becoming energized.

---

[7] A pioneer in the field, Andrew Newberg, M.D., neuroscientist from the University of Pennsylvania and Director of Research at the Myrna Brind Center for Integrative Medicine (Thomson Jefferson University Hospital and Medical College) has been scanning brains for over a decade.

Normally random number generators give us a consistent run of the mill, random, sequence of numbers in zeroes and 1's. During highly charged or impactful world events in which a collective energy is emitted from all areas of the globe (i.e. 9/11, the death of Princess Diana, the World Series, global soccer events, etc.), we see these numbers change quite remarkably in their sequence, notably indicating there is a connection in the energy or thought we are emitting into the Universe.

During sad events we can feel the energy of others even when they are far away. During happy events you can feel it, the electricity buzzing and filling the atmosphere. The thoughts within our minds impact more than what is inside of us individually, we are outputting our energy to the collective consciousness of the Universe. We are entangled in each other's energy, and energy of the Source. Regardless of what you call that Source, or if you do not believe in one at all, doesn't matter. The power of prayer enhances your experience and your path, it does not validate it.

When I think about prayer, I think about the old saying, *"God helps those that help themselves."* In other words, when we pray the idea is not to ask for Him to deliver the goods, but to ask for strength in order to obtain the thing we want by our own means, our own actions, or our own struggle. Just as if we wouldn't pray for a new car to show up the next morning in the driveway, (instead, we might pray for a good job or the ability to save money) we wouldn't pray for world peace without praying for the strength to stop judging others, asking for the ability to forgive, or requesting that He make you an instrument of peace. Praying is about hope and strength; it is about wanting to be the best you can be and doing the best you can do. Praying should be done daily. Religions and philosophies, when practiced correctly, that is according to divine nature – The Golden Rule for example, and through self-control, charity, pure mind, forgiveness, truth, freedom, non-judgment, detachment from anger, fear, jealousy, and above all *love for all.* When practiced correctly, these embodiments soothe the spirit and elevate the soul consciousness. Almost every faith holds sacred mysteries which are always conveyed through one God, in three states of beings.[8]

---

[8] Including but not limited to: *Sumeria*: Anu (ruler of heaven), Ea (ruler of water), and Enlil (ruler of Earth); *Hindu:* Brahma (Creates), Vishnu (Maintains), and Shiva (destroys so that rejuvenation can take place); *Christian*: Father, Son, Holy Ghost; *Egyptian*: Amun, Re, and Ptah as well as others such as Osiris, Isis, and Horus, or Amen, Mut, and Khonsu; *Phoenician*: Ulomus, Ulosuros, and Eliun; *Greek*: Zeus, Poseiden, and Adonis; *Buddhist*: three bodies of enlightenment - Dharmakaya (body of ultimate reality), Sambhogakaya (body of joy), and Nirmanakaya (body of flesh and blood) and also Amitabha the Buddha of Infinite Life and Life (represented by the trio: Amida, Amita, Amitayus*); Wicca*: Goddess, God, and Dryghten.

Most commonly thought of as a Christian belief, the concept of trinity is actually a very ancient belief held by almost all civilizations in our history. What this tells us is that since records have been kept, we all believe in something Divine, something higher, something outside of ourselves that is just as much a part of us as our physical self, and actually even greater. It tells us that life continues after death.

Meditation

"The real point of meditation is to rest
in bare awareness whether anything occurs or not.
Whatever comes up for you, just be open
and present to it, and let it go.
And if nothing occurs, or if thoughts and so on
vanish before you can notice them,
just rest in that natural clarity."[9]
Yongey Mingyur Rinpoche

Meditation allows us to go to a quiet space within, and relax in the space between thoughts. It is the most peaceful level of consciousness and provides your body with deep rest. Think of it this way, meditation is to the mind, what massage is to the body. Meditation is not at all difficult and it is beneficial to all ages. Surrounded by peace, this is a sacred time between you and Source - between you and cosmic love.

---

[9] Yongey Mingyur Rinpoche is a Buddhist teacher and author of *The Joy of Living: Unlocking the Secret & Science of Happiness*. Quote from page 131.

There are a few different ways to meditate and the method you decide on is merely personal preference. If you are just beginning to learn, I would recommend a guided meditation whereas you will listen to a CD which will guide you visually into a meditative state.

It is a fact that meditation benefits the mind and body. I believe if everyone knew a little about the science behind the brain and meditation, more people would practice meditation on a daily basis. Let's discuss some basics about what happens to the brain during meditation. There are several areas in the brain which have different jobs and functions, but we'll concentrate on those that are important in understanding the importance of meditation.

The lateral prefrontal cortex (Assessment Center) is the area of the brain that gives us balance in the way we look at things. It's where our perspective, reasoning ability, and logic reside.

The insula is responsible for our intuitional or gut feelings and works also with the part of the Me Center (next page) in the ability to feel compassion and empathy.

The amygdala (Fear Center) gives us our fight-or-flight reactions and is where our initial emotions originate.

The medial prefrontal cortex ("Me" Center) processes information related to you, thus the Me Center. Within the Me Center we find two areas that are very strongly connected and work together because of the strength of the neural paths connecting them:

The first is a place that processes information related to you such as anxiety, worry, and depression. The second place is where we process information about people we see as differently from ourselves. It's where compassion and empathy, for instance, come from.

Due to the way our brains function naturally, there is a weak neural connection between our assessment center and the Me Center, which is why we sometimes get stuck in a thought, feeling, or emotion. It's the reason we tell ourselves repetitive stories, or harp on the feelings of being ill. The weak connection is the reason we linger on our mistakes and problems and obsess about how we are feeling.

Meditation helps the connections between the Me Center and the Fear Center break down, while at the same time helps the connections between the Me Center and the Assessment Center build up. In a nutshell what this means is through meditation we can control our pain, anxiety, and fear, as well as experience compassion and empathy toward others. Meditation pretty much helps our brain to balance. Imagine if we all practiced meditation on a daily basis.

Meditation is as important to our mind and body as vitamins and minerals are. Issues and problems become easier to handle as you understand your ability to let them go. Meditation increases happiness, calm, intuition, creativity, clarity, sharpness, breathing, the ability to pay attention, and the ability to relax on will. It improves the immune system, energy levels, and increases serotonin. At the same time meditation decreases stress, anxiety, anger, frustration, and tension. Regular practice will lower blood pressure, tension, pain levels, the ability to focus, and will boost your memory.

Meditation also is very helpful for your gray matter! There is a documented increase in gray matter in meditating individuals along with stronger cognitive abilities that normally weaken upon aging.

The practice of meditation generally will have you focusing on something, such as the flame of a candle, a mantra, a beat, or your breath. There are also certain postures to successful meditation sessions. It is completely normal to experience a bombardment of thoughts when you meditate. They may flood your mind similar to a bad night sleep – only it feels like you are tossing and turning while awake. When this happens you want to acknowledge the thought (it is here, I see it) and let it go, bringing yourself back to focusing on your breath or whatever it was you used to start your meditation. Keep in mind that getting upset with yourself for having these thoughts or thinking that you're doing it wrong – is what is hindering your session because that is what you are now focusing on. So it is not the thoughts cropping up which are disturbing you – it is your reaction to the thoughts. This is why you acknowledge the thought and then let it go and bring your focus back.

Through practice, you will find that not only during meditation, but in everyday life, you will be better able to see your thought, feeling, emotion, situation or issue, and attend to it without over reacting, and let it go. Meditation will free your mind. In order for these benefits you must practice it often, even daily.

You may not notice the full effects of meditation (other than feeling amazing and being fully rested) immediately. It will take some time of regular practice. The calm and relaxed state are beautiful bi-product of a much deeper goal – which is to be able to get to the root of your feelings, thoughts, and emotions and deal with them in a healthy manner; to investigate why you think and feel certain ways; to make adjustments to those ways – allowing a more balanced and healthier mind.

The Four Virtues

Virtues are our behaviors which define good moral values. They are useful traits that give us good character.

Over 2500 years ago, Lao Tzu gave us the *Tao te Ching*. The now ancient texts serve as a roadmap to millions of souls worldwide. It is through the Tao which we learn the four principal virtues. These four virtues help us to develop additional virtues such as trust, patience, understanding, authenticity, commitment, compassion, faith, ethics, grace, fairness, honesty, humility, perseverance, strength, justice, modesty, responsibility, reliability, tolerance, wisdom, unity, and many more. As we apply our virtues, we strengthen our virtues.

1. Reverence for All Life

When we conduct our lives with the understanding that we all come from one Source, we develop reverence for all living things. All life deserves, and should be treated with, respect. Although we all conduct our lives in a different manner from one another, although we physically look different, practice different religions, or behave differently – putting all this aside – we are all of one Source. Therefore, we honor all life without judgment and critical assessment and we love all life unconditionally because all life comes from the Divine. We must also keep in mind that we, ourselves, are

69

included in this. To love one's self is foundation for loving all others. To be in harmony with all life is truly the only way to discover divine love.

2. Sincerity

When we are sincere, we are also honest. Perhaps the simplest and most important of all virtues – sincerity is one of the most difficult to practice. It's about practicing what you preach and living authentically.

3. Gentleness

When we accept people for who they are, just as they are, without conditions, and without wanting them to be something they simply are not – we give up control over always needing to be right. Cherishing someone as they are rather who we think they should be. We become compassionate, considerate, and gentle.

4. Supportiveness

When we stop focusing on ourselves and make the Ego take the back seat, we find our greatest gift is that of service to others. When we support each other regardless of outward appearance or circumstance, we grow spiritually. The moment you decide someone is beneath you, the moment you feel you are the bigger or better person, is the moment you dishonor your soul. The virtue of supportiveness is an integral part on the path to enlightenment.

These Four Virtues remind me of the teachings of Jesus. In Galatians 5:22-23 Paul writes, *"But the fruit of the Spirit is love, joy, peace, forbearance, kindness, goodness, faithfulness, gentleness and self-control. Against such things there is no law."*

Embracing Connection

The whole concept of spiritual awakening begins with connection – connection to your sense of self, connection to Source (the Divine, the Universe, the Sacred), and a connection to all living things. We experience connection through our senses, our relationships, through faith, and through nature. We deepen those connections when we are able to see beyond that which is first visible to our eyes.

When we are able to experience life deeper than the materialistic level and find worth and purpose in all that surrounds us (good and bad), we grow spiritually. The first step is embracing yourself and loving yourself as you are right now. Taking out of the equation all the things you wish you were, or weren't, and being thankful for all that you actually are. When we embrace nature we delve into the beauty of creation itself and practice a deep appreciation for the beautiful world in which we live in.

In other words, if you are serving dinner and you scoop up a serving of potatoes, you're not just thankful for the potato you are grateful and amazed by all the factors that went into that potato winding up on your plate. Go backwards and appreciate the farmer that tended, nurtured, and harvested the potato, be thankful for the sun and rain, the soil, and the root that slept below the ground.

When you look at a flower, imagine constant life force moving within it. From seed to blossom how it has grown and thrived to provide your eyes with beauty, your nose with fragrance, or your world with medicinal value. Sit and listen to the sound of a stream – the delightful, calming sensation that consumes you as you tune out everything around you except the water. Imagine following the stream backwards to the land source, up to the clouds, and back down to where it originated from. Capture your feelings and insight in a creative way, such as photography, writing, song, or art.

Embrace the connections you have with others by allowing them to be themselves and loving them just the way they are. Be open and receptive to differences in culture, language, class, and religion. Close your eyes and imagine the energy, the breath, flowing in and flowing out of your body – the breath which circulates knowing no boundaries between these differences, having no distinction between any forms of life.

A greater appreciation for all life develops once we embrace these connections. We can then truly understand the words *We Are One* and begin to make an impact globally.

Be Brave

It's not about wanting something better in life it is about being grateful and enjoying what you have on your plate right now. To do this you must be brave and deal with whatever comes your way. When I was growing up I hated peas. The thought of them made me shudder, but I was required to have a spoonful of peas on my plate when peas were being served. I'd hem and haw over those peas. They always got cold as I pushed them around my plate hoping they would magically disappear. First I tried hiding them under the mashed potatoes, but my crime was foiled and I was told I would have to finish everything on my plate. Then I began to spit them in a small amount of milk in my glass when no one was looking. Foiled again, the next time I was instructed to finish the last gulp before leaving the table. I could hear the neighborhood kids laughing and playing while I pushed those damned peas.

The point is, we can avoid the peas in life, but eventually we must confront them. Deal with your issues at the moment. You'll end up learning that what your mind cooked up as an impossible task – is not impossible at all. Plow through the difficult things in life, and when you look back you'll find it wasn't as bad as you thought it would be. Be brave. Do what you have to do in order to resolve issues and move forward.

6.

Good, Good, Good,
Good Vibrations

Everything is made up of energy. Every single cell gives off energy and disperses it outward, so energy is always in motion, it's vibrating. If you look at a burning candle, you can see the energy radiating from the wick. Everything radiates energy – it is just that sometimes we can't see it. Basically, as we go through life, our energy is making direct contact with everybody else's energy around us. Think of drops of colored water dripped onto a piece of paper. The droplets spread out and bump into, mesh, and weave together with the other droplets.

Now think about this for a moment because so many things begin to make complete sense when you do. This clearly explains why when we are in a room and someone is negative or feeling down – everyone feels it. Or when we spend time with positive people – we feel positive too. All that vibrating energy is branching out and touching everyone else's energy!

Each of us is made up of over 75 trillion cells. Each cell is vibrating, and everyone's cells vibrate at a different speed or frequency. When your cells are vibrating faster you are healthier; when they vibrate slowly you are not feeling well. Happiness, laughter, positive thinking, being in love, expressing compassion — all these things make our cells vibrate fast and make us feel great! When our cells are happy — we are happy. When our cells are healthy — we are healthy. It really is that simple!

When we experience negativity, sickness, depression, anger, jealousy, and disease – these things make our cells vibrations get slower. We become more negative, depressed, and drained physically or mentally. When our cells are vibrating slower, we can become sick — in mind and body.

Now that you are armed with knowledge about your vibrating cells, you can use this to become mentally and physically healthy! Eat healthy so that your cells don't feel sluggish. Think and act positively: Surround yourself with positive people, find the positive in situations, and participate in positive physical activities (such as walking, biking, laughing, gardening, or any form of exercise.)

When you find yourself absorbing negative energy you must remove yourself from the situation by walking away, or turning your attention to something positive! Whether it's your boss, your eye-rolling teenager, or that friend who came in holding a big can of drama in one hand and a can opener in the other hand – turn your attention to positive thoughts or you will certainly be sucked into having a negative day.

Yoga, prayer, and meditation all affect us at our core – our vibrational level. Practice one or all of them daily.

Chorus of Souls

7.

Arriving Souls

Ancient philosophies teach us that we choose our parents. The choice is made according to who will provide an atmosphere or avenue conducive to achieving our soul mission. The soul will incarnate into the circumstances it feels best fit the lessons it needs to learn, as well as the lessons it needs to teach. So, you might pick loving parents, you might pick dysfunction, you might choose someone who gives you away to another couple, and you might select someone who doesn't want you at all.

When I hear people say, "If choosing your parents were true – why on Earth would I have chosen the parents I have?" I say it is because you knew before you were born that you needed to accomplish certain things (whether easy or difficult, happy or sad) in order to further your divine training. You knew way ahead of time who you were choosing, and what you were striving for. You knew you could handle it – it is just that you forgot inside your human mind and body. You came here knowing, but through human conditioning, your upbringing, and your environment, you forgot that purpose and became sidetracked living humanly rather than divinely. Have faith in yourself – your soul's purpose guided you to this life.

One might wonder, if I chose my own life ahead of time, why did I choose such a difficult one? Your soul knows that to understand the lesson and to grow to be divine, it needs to use the human form – the body and mind and it's multiple senses – to experience life and work through those lessons. It will choose the avenue it feels best to educate its self. Also, keep in mind that just because someone else's life looks easy, everyone is going through their own learning process. You can be the richest person on Earth and have all the finest things and still not understand what it means to truly love and to live through your soul. On the other hand, you might be struggling your whole life and still possess the ability to find compassion for everyone. The soul doesn't select their journey based on money or fame, it chooses the best avenue in which to learn and experience.

This is why, no matter what sort of obstacle you face, you should understand that everything is happening for a reason. There is purpose in each and every day. There is opportunity to embrace your life and your journey. When you accomplish this, the journey is a bit easier because you are not hindered by the thought that you've been dealt a bad hand – because you know your soul selected this hand – your task is now to figure out what you can do with it and make the most of it.

We need conflict in order to progress. Through conflict we experience growth. Without growth the soul will not advance. Once you embrace yourself, accept your life, figure out what to do with it, and rediscover your authentic self, you will gain confidence and start opening up that direct path between your soul and home. This will allow the flow of the divine to work through you, to heal you, to make you stronger. Within your authentic self you will discover more compassion and love and how to properly extend those gifts to all others regardless of how your "humanness" may have tempted you to judge. Souls come in imprinted with who they were in their last life and with an accumulated karma which has not yet been paid or collected upon. Souls come in when they are ready, just as they leave when they are ready. Arriving at the moment of conception, as the egg unites with the sperm, the soul becomes a sentient being[10].

The time spent in gestation soothes, protects and calms you for the journey you are about to embark on. Although you are not predestined to a specific way you

---

[10] Sentience (or consciousness) refers to the ability to feel, perceive and process, experience pain, and to suffer. Sentient beings encompass all living things which include, but are not limited to, humans and animals.

81

will travel along your path, you do know the lessons you are supposed to learn and overcome during your time in this life. The life you choose to be reborn into is relative to the lessons you must learn. You are also well aware of what you will teach others in your time here.

After the soul arrives and enters the Earth realm with its first breath, many things start happening. We have parents and siblings, there are many loved ones surrounding us. Over time, we develop friendships, and relationships which either nurture us or cause us pain. All of the things that we brought with us from the space between death and life are slowly tucked away and become replaced with layers and layers of learned behaviors, thoughts, and beliefs of those around us. Eventually we have a deep desire to shed those layers and find the seed of knowledge that we came here bearing.

We discover this sacred seed to be swaddled in our spirituality. We now need to relearn how to use the tools we arrived here with. We need to understand karma and how it works. This knowledge provides a beneficial environment in which to begin your journey.

8.

Departing Souls

Souls enter and exit when they are ready. It is normal to feel sadness upon loss but we must look upon death as it is way down to the core: the soul has finished its work here. It accomplished what it needed to and has returned home – as we all will – and will return again when it is time to receive another lesson, or engage in continued divine training. Some souls are here for a very brief moment – a mere snap of the fingers in what we would consider to be a lifetime. The little ones who we feel leave us too soon – leaving behind crushed parents with broken hearts and shattered dreams. The souls who go home in what seems to be the prime of their Earthly lives – leaving us shocked and bewildered, and the souls who stay in their human form for many years.

The truth of the matter is we should all rejoice for these departing loved ones! Of course we will feel our emotions from loss on the Earthly level (we are human at the time after all). Our hearts will ache, break, we will cry and we will mourn. Grief is a normal and healthy process that we must invite and experience. As humans we are

83

not equipped to experience loss without pain. There is no time limit on grief and everyone experiences it in different ways, but we must push through grief by allowing the experience and the emotions. If we do not – we will be stuck in it. We must remember at the core of it all – death is so much bigger than the Earthly experience. That soul came here specifically to do something – to give something – to receive something – to learn something – or to teach something. It arrived as love and returned as love. Love is the memory that must be celebrated. The soul should be remembered at death in the same way it was remembered at birth. It entered the physical world bearing gifts. This soul chose to be a part of your life; it chose to deliver a gift to you. This gift was a special delivery from a divine place.

To remain stuck – to remain prisoner to grief and sadness – does not honor the journey of that departed soul. To remember the anniversary of a death immersed in sadness or to grieve about what that loved one would be doing today had they lived – is a sad way to celebrate a soul because that soul was ready to go home. It was their time no matter how tragic or soon the death. Departed souls do not want your sadness, they want your love and understanding of what they presented you with during the time they were with you. They don't want you to wallow in pain. Dwell upon the gift they have brought to you while they were here, rather than the loss of the personality you knew.

Though the millions of near death stories from all corners of the globe, and from the teachings of Eastern philosophies, we clearly understand that dying is both a beautiful and confusing time for the transitioning soul. Much in the way we enter a new body upon arrival, from the intermediate space between death and rebirth, the soul must get its bearings back upon physical death in order to move forward and begin its journey once again. The majority of religions and philosophies, both ancient and modern, hold the belief that all our souls, spirits, or our streams of consciousness reincarnate multiple times. The form in which your soul will reside – human, animal, plant, etc.) is based on your karma and moral behavior in the present life – the quality of our choices and actions.

Those with near death experiences recount a darkness followed by a brilliant white light – brighter than many suns – to which the soul gravitates. We learn of a reunion with the souls that went ahead of us and an experience of a visual life review from the life we just came from. When the consciousness departs the body permanently the human form is dead. Rituals are performed on the body of the deceased while the consciousness travels to that intermediate divine space between life and death. Imprinted upon your consciousness is your karma. Karma boils down to all the good and all the bad you had accumulated during the life you left, and you will be taking that all along with you to the place after death. The ratio of good karma (debt owed to you) and bad karma (debt owed to others) will be a huge factor in determining where your soul (or consciousness) will end up in the next rebirth. It should also be noted that good and bad karma do not cancel either other out. It's not as if you have in one hand 500 good deeds and the other hand 500 bad deeds, so that would wipe the slate clean. It doesn't work that way.

Having more good karma than bad will land back into human form, while more bad than good will get you the form of an animal, for instance. And, upon each death you can fall into any of these levels *regardless of the places you have incarnated before.* Throughout your lives and experiences, the rebirth cycle can be broken by paying your karmic debt in full without accumulating further debt. According to many philosophies the human and animal realms are only two of the several realms you can end up in, and all these give us the nature of suffering – just in varying degrees.

Another key note in where you end up in the next rebirth depends upon the state of mind you are in at the time of death. We want our being to be of a positive mind; to be filled with compassion, love, happiness, and calm. If, at the time of death, the person is conscious they can pray, meditate and reflect upon their life. If unconscious, someone can help them by praying or meditating with (or for) them. Remember – if someone is unconscious it does not mean they cannot hear you and it does not mean they cannot feel or understand you. It is critical that those departing have some guidance and remain focused on the positive, remain calm, and stay happy for their journey ahead. Regardless of the consciousness or unconsciousness at the time of death, we can help those souls by praying with them, encouraging thoughts of positive, of love, of calm, and by giving them compassion. These things can be done aloud or silently and they should continue to be done daily for about a month after they have departed.

Buddhist tradition, for example, teaches us that the departed can hear us, feel us, and are still receptive to our thoughts for nearly a month after dying. They still have a connection of consciousness to us. So talk to them, pray for them, and encourage calm and happiness. Wish them well along their journey, thank them for all they have taught you, and instruct them to enter the white light. Remember, you will see them again. Your souls will reunite again when it is time.

We find the idea of positive, calming departure of souls in many religions. We hold ceremonies for the departed in whichever way that particular religion practices. It might be good, at the time of death, to have something visually calming in the room such as an image of a religious figure that was important in their life. Consider though, that it should be something or someone important in their life, in their belief (not yours if it is not the same). If the idea is for them to remain calm you wouldn't want to, for instance, have a big Buddha in the room if they themselves followed Jesus (or vice versa).

While the manner of death oftentimes adds to our grief, if it's tragic or unexpected especially, those left behind must remember the soul departing was ready to leave. However sad and rooted in pain you feel over the loss – it is imperative to understand the importance of love, and calm encouragement as the soul continues its journey. Suicide, for example, is a very hard way to leave, on both the departing soul as well as the people it leaves behind.

Considering the frame of mind at death, it will be a more trying transition, and in the same way as we create karma from everything else we experience in life, the suffering of this life will be brought to the next.

Regardless of the manner of death we can begin to understand the importance of working through our issues, obstacles, and experiences which we encounter during our lifetimes.

9.

Healing a Sick Soul

Sometimes along the way in our personal journey, maybe even several times in a lifetime, our soul might become sick. The symptoms present themselves in a few key ways. You might start out sensing there is something you should be doing but cannot quite put your finger on it. You may start to sense the direction you are heading in doesn't feel right.

You might feel of unappreciated or as if you've lost your sense of self. This is very common among parents, especially mothers, who devote their time to raising their children while neglecting themselves in the process. We have to learn that while our children mean the world to us, it is imperative to the development of the child to be raised by a parent with a healthy mind and soul. Too many of us fail to allow ourselves some personal time and space to develop, grow, and maintain a healthy inner self. When the parent feels negative the corrupt energy will be absorbed by the child. Pretending to be positive with an underlying negative feeling is just as bad. A child can sense when something is off or wrong and then they are just plain confused. They pick up on everything no matter how hard you try to hide it or pretend that everything is all sunshine and roses.

When your soul is sick, sometimes the way it expresses itself is through the body, sometimes through the mind, and sometimes through both. You've heard it said so many times, *"You don't have a soul. You are a soul. You have a body, temporarily.[11]"* Well, I can tell you from personal experience that when your soul is sick and it's not corrected in a timely fashion, the only way for your soul to scream out that it needs help – is to make the body ill. Sometimes the mind is so confused that it doesn't realize the behavior you are engaging in is wrong, therefore the soul, with its pent up energy, is itching to correct itself and manifests as a sick body. It could be something as simple as chronic headaches, unusual acne outbreaks, or stomach ailments. Left unattended it could result in disease. When the soul manifests its discomfort using the mind, you could experience confusion, depression, or mental illness.

Every now and then in life, we find ourselves with a sick soul. Things feel off, our lives feel topsy-turvy, life feels as if we're living according to Murphy's Law. We might have taken ill or feel depressed. A sick soul can,

---

[11] Walter M. Miller, Jr., *A Canticle for Leibowitz*, 1960.

and usually will, happen to everyone. It can last any length of time, depending on how your react to situations and people, and what actions you take to heal your soul.

Finding the root of your woes, the source of your pain is very important. When you hear people saying "Think positive," they are correct – you should. But, you first must experience and feel the source of your pain, anger, jealousy, addiction, loneliness, or whatever it is that is causing your grief. You cannot simply push aside these thoughts, feelings and experiences and not deal with them. If you don't deal with your self-destructive behavior you are simply avoiding the source of your sick soul. The source, if not dealt with, will rear its ugly head at any chance it gets and will keep making your life miserable, as well as hindering your personal journey.

None of the things that you are experiencing happened with the snap of a finger, therefore they are not going to go away with a snap of a finger. It takes time to heal your soul; it takes time to turn around. Allow yourself the time to feel your own pain. When you struggle, when you are in pain, anger, addiction, jealousy or loneliness, these struggles will consume you. (They will cause you to feel crazy, act badly, and become desperate.) You will become a snowball of negative emotion rolling and rolling down a cliff, gathering more negative energy as you fall. As a result, you will become physically and mentally weakened. You will find yourself seeking like-minded negative people to reinforce how awful life is. You will feed off their stories and hunger to share your own with them. As you tell yourself how unjust the world is to you, it becomes more so because you are constantly thinking, believing, living and attracting this negativity. By choosing to remain in this energy – you have requested more of it from the Universe. Some might say, "Choose to remain here? I don't choose to remain here!" I would ask them what they are doing to change. I would ask them what they have learned from their experiences. What are they taking away from their troubles? When you feel life has dealt you a bad hand you must find a way to play that hand so that you can turn your circumstances around. And, the hand must be played using the gifts you cradle within yourself: compassion, patience, love, gratitude, and grace.

It is only when you come to the conclusion that you need to break out, when you understand that you do have a problem, that you are at the point in which you are ready to begin the healing process.

So what now? You are standing at the bottom of the mountain with your hiking gear on, ready to make the journey to the summit. First, understand there are many paths before you all leading to the same place. The degree of difficulty along your path at any given time will

94

vary, but you must remain committed and strong. You must keep moving along.

With the first step taken, understand that you will be responsible for everything that you will create and everything you have already created. Understand in your heart that you alone are responsible for your own value and worth, that acceptance must come from within, and that at this very moment you are divine love. You are worthy, you are of value, and you are love right now because you are a sentient being. It is not a matter of one day being or having these things – you are these things now no matter what situation you are in at the time. You were born of the divine and are already equipped with the tools you need to heal yourself. Let's begin.

Words

"Your beliefs become your thoughts,

Your thoughts become your words,

Your words become your actions,

Your actions become your habits,

Your habits become your values,

Your values become your destiny."

Mahatma Gandhi

Be careful how you use your words. When you speak, even when you think, you are sending words out – words with far reaching tentacles; words which travel to God, the Universe; words which reach out and touch everyone around you. Your thoughts and words, not unlike your actions, become energy and affect you, they affect everyone around you, and they become the life you bring to yourself. Cease the spewing of negative words, thoughts, and emotions.

Instead of telling God and the Universe how unhappy you are, begin to tell the tale of how grateful you are for what you do have at this moment. From playing a sport to completing a project, from taking a test to being in a relationship – if you keep telling yourself you stink at something, if you keep acknowledging how awful you are doing – what you are actually projecting is that you are not good enough, you are reinforcing (to yourself, the Universe, and everyone around you) that you simply are not worthy of success or happiness. That which you project outward will be that which you draw back toward you.

Never, ever, ever speak negative words. Not about yourself, or about anyone else. They hinder your spiritual growth and they attract negative back to you. Try your absolute best to think about the line you are casting out there and what you are inevitably going to reel back in. Even if you feel it deep within you – start replacing those negative words with positive affirmations. It takes time and a lot of practice, but when you feel the negative words touching your lips, stop! Substitute something positive instead.

I AM beautiful. I AM confident. I AM worthy. Practice your own positive I AMs on a regular basis.

Courage

We know our goal is to work through life using compassion, love, grace, and patience. Although we already have all these core values, these virtues, deep within ourselves, through the years of being reconditioned during our human upbringing, we have forgotten how to practice and implement them, as we should have been using them all along. We selectively practice these virtues when we should be freely giving them away to all. In order to do this we must develop courage. This is a big step for many as oftentimes it requires us to step outside of our comfort zone. We develop courage by taking baby steps. It's no different than the way we approach other difficult things in our life. When we want to get physically fit we don't begin by going out and immediately running a marathon – we start by beginning an appropriate exercise program for beginners – and eating healthy.

Be Authentic

Be clear about boundaries and values. Stand firm, tall, and remain clear about them. Trust in your ability to stay strong. Stop laughing at the off-color jokes, refrain from smiling in uncomfortable situations because you don't want to go against the norm, and when you hear an untruth – you must find your voice and stand up for what is right. Too many times we overlook the negative in life because we want it to go away. Rather than taking a stand, we remain complacent. Over time, we continue to hear the off-color remarks, we continue to remain in the room with the half-wits, and we continue to sit with our heads lowered – fearful of voicing our own authentic self. The result is living with shame and thus reinforcing the negative things we had hoped to tackle in the first place.

When we express ourselves from our heart, when we unshackle our authentic self, when we take that stand, and speak our love for all – we trigger something within us. Our spirit receives a spark. Adrenaline floods our system and we feel great! Sometimes we get shaky from the burst of adrenaline as it rushes throughout our body and brain. The natural high is as if the Universe has embraced us, we feel wonderful, and aligned. Letting go of what other people think of you is a huge step into liberating your soul. It is the one major step you will take in the journey to discovering your authentic self.

99

Feel and Understand

Thinking you will put your problems aside, not visit them, and they will go away is about as easy as setting aside your favorite dessert while dieting, and trying to stop your mouth from watering. It is not possible. In order to heal yourself you have to look at what is going on. You must feel what is going on inside your body. How does it make you feel? Where in your body do you feel this? How does it manifest within your body? Do these feelings, this situation, these thoughts give you headaches, stomach aches, or create a sense of sadness within you? Do you experience insomnia, addiction, or depression as a result of your feelings? Are you drowning in a cesspool of shame or suffering?

The only way you will be able to get through your pain is to literally go through your pain. Let your feelings out and talk about them. Holding in your thoughts, emotions, fears, negative feelings will only foster further suffering; harboring these things causes physical and mental pain.

Understand that your own shame and suffering should never be compared to anyone else's shame and suffering. Just because so-in-so is going through this or that and it seems bigger than what is happening to you – does not make your own shame and suffering any less important. Talk about your issues, bring them forward and let them out. You cannot look at anyone else's situation or plight and feel as if your own issues are less (or more) important. If you are experiencing hurt, anger, jealousy, pain, addiction, etc. you must allow yourself to find the root and fix the problem. If you do not allow this experience, you will stew and stew until you are beyond overcooked.

Tell your story to those you trust. Do not seek out those who are going to enable your bad behavior, do not yearn for those that are going to agree with you no matter what. Pass by the friends that want to fix it for you or who map out a scenario of what you should do next complete with a script and a timetable. Search for someone who is going to close their mouth and let you speak. Rejoice in the one who passes no judgment but instead takes your hand and says, "I am here for you." Be thankful for the friend who doesn't want to remove your burden for you, but is willing to hold your hand while you remove it for yourself.

Energy is constantly flowing into and out of our body. It is a system not unlike our circulatory system or any of the systems that keep us functioning. Energy from all around us filters in to us. It is processed into emotion, such as love, compassion, patience, anger, jealousy, frustration, etc., and the energy is released from our body. We all receive the same energy in pure form, but it is the way in which we individually process the energy that determines the emotion it becomes.

The way humans process energy can be compared to the way a group of people experience a meadow. Flowers are in full bloom, the wind is creating a gentle breeze, and pollen is dancing visibly in the air. Some of the people in the group will sneeze uncontrollably, some intermittently, some not at all. Some people are allergic to one variety of flower, others are allergic to a different flower. Some are allergic to the grass, and others are sensitive to the tree pollen. Everyone has the same processing system, they function in the same way, but how they process within that system is very much unique. The same applies for people with food allergies or intolerance and the digestive system. Similarly, the air we breathe and our circulatory system. In order to control, maintain, or alleviate these issues within our systems, we might use medications, herbs, some form of treatment, or watch our diet. When you have an allergic reaction it is your body speaking to you. It says "This item needs attention!"

Energy systems are a bit different. When we experience emotions they stem from our energy processing. It is not our body speaking, *but our soul.* It is saying, "This item needs attention!" To adjust our energy systems we must look within ourselves and understand why it is we are turning this energy into the negative (or positive) emotion.

To do this you have to really take some time daily and think about your energy and emotions. What sensations do you have in your body, and where do you feel these sensations within your body? Have you felt these feelings before and did they manifest the same sensations in the same places? How you process your energy is rooted in all that you have learned, and how you have been conditioned to process that energy. If you study your emotions you will find they are deeply rooted in either fear or love. Negative emotions are rooted in fear; positive emotions in love. So, you may find, for instance, the anger or jealousy you feel about a current situation is rooted in a trust issue, and the trust issue is rooted in a situation you experienced in your formative years which caused you fear – fear of what might happen next, fear of loss, fear of whatever. Once you learn where these current ways of processing energy are coming from, and you understand that you do not have to process energy in that way any longer. You can choose to simply acknowledge the emotion as it comes up and decide to process it differently, because it is no longer about the past and seeing that feeling as fear – it is now about making a conscious decision to process the energy in a positive way.

Let me give you a personal example: I had always been a people pleaser. I really didn't want discourse and a tense atmosphere, so I would end up doing things to ensure a happy medium around me. I would attend family functions even though I knew I would be uncomfortable and unhappy. As a child of divorce entering a new paternal family with some of those family members not quite accepting of the situation, I entered into a tense situation. Never were their comments or words directly outwardly to me personally, but I could feel the energy released and it was obviously strained and negative.

As I grew up with very loving parents, my mom and my adoptive dad, things were wonderful on the home front. It was bringing in the extended family that became an issue for me. Although I came to love many of them dearly, there were a few that could simply ruin a function for me. I would come home feeling confused, drained, and hurt. Again, it wasn't anything they said outright – more like in the way they carried themselves, mannerisms, and how they came across.

I started to dread family functions, but I didn't want to disappoint this person or that person, even at the risk of making myself miserable, so I would attend. It was a process that repeated itself for many years. One day I decided to really look at how I was feeling. I found I didn't like how I was feeling. The thought of being with these people made my stomach upset and my mind crazy. I thought ahead of time how I would react and what I might say. I held conversations in my mind with myself coming out the winner – finally saying the things I have always wanted to express. Of course, that never happened in person.

I decided I was going to remove myself from the offending situation and stop the way I was allowing myself to feel. I was now fully aware of where this emotion was coming from and I knew there were a couple things I could choose to do. I could go to the function with the advance understanding that my buttons might be pushed – allowing myself to be ready, feel the experience and immediately let it go. I would tell myself, *"This is how they are. I can get up and leave at any time. I will not let their attitude determine how I feel the rest of the day;"* I could fly off the handle and speak my mind – creating more tension, or I could stay home and avoid the situation all together. For the next few family functions, I choose the first option and this became the point of my personal journey. Once I understood fully that it was me, it was how *I processed* the energy in my life that created how I felt and thought, I was better able to move forward into a healthier life. I was eventually able to choose the option of not attending at all, because through working on my inner self I learned I was not attending to avoid the situation, but because I valued my time and fully understood I did not have to subject myself to negative. Had I avoided the function as my first choice, I would have never learned the importance of detachment.

Eventually, with practice, I could trace my feelings backward even further to my biological father – the mental and physical abuse he dealt to my mom, and the resulting divorce. I found all sorts of ways I currently process energy – from trust issues to acceptance issues and many more. I took a step back and looked deeper. Some of these trust and acceptance issues were prevalent in my family. I started to see repeating patterns.

Then it hit me – these are lessons I have been sent here to learn. This is the karma from another life that I must work through. My problems *are not a result* of my childhood; my childhood was simply the way my soul selected to work through my karma. The situations presented to me since childhood were the earliest beginnings of these lessons; they were the most conducive environment for the growth of my soul.

We all possess that Sacred Seed which contains everything we need along our journey through life. While we were in gestation, preparing for our new life within the comfort of the womb, the seed stood by idly. With our first breath, we immediately forgot much of our previous lives. We now had family and friends who would consciously or unconsciously guide us through actions or words around our new world. Their actions and words are a reflection of the tools they have unlocked within their own Sacred Seed at the point they were in during their own life. They were doing the best they knew how to do at that time, in the place they were in, and with the tools they had unlocked. We cannot fault those we took our cues from any more than we can fault our child-self for not having cracked open the seed early on. The circumstances of this life came as a result of everyone working out their own previous karma. It is up to each of us individually to dig deep, find our spiritual tools, and navigate these situations with pure love and light.

Such an eye opening and liberating revelation! It is not our parents or our childhood that mess up our lives – we are messed up, because over the years, the lessons have not been learned! All these things have taken place to help us, not hurt us. Knowing this helps us to stop blaming others and shoulder the responsibility of our own way of thinking.

Sometimes we are given quite a harsh lesson as a child or as an adult. Experiences that carry lasting pain. Some of these should be worked through with the help of a professional. There is no shame in seeking help, it will only aid in your healing process.

Letting go of the root situation will greatly benefit the processing of energy and emotions in the present. But don't be fooled! Looking at your emotions and feeling what they are doing within you and to you is not a one-time deal. It is not as if you do it once and you're fixed. It is a work in progress, like fighting an addiction. The good thing is when you have learned how to detach, how to let it go, it becomes easier as you go along and practice the process. You will get to a point where you are able to see the feeling, experience it, and release it before it consumes you.

"Let Go or Be Dragged."

Zen Proverb

How to Detach

Any feeling that binds you to another person, thing, cause, ideal, or feeling – is attachment. In my last book, *Booyah! Spirit*, I talked about the process of detaching.

Figure out who or what causes you grief.

Look at why you have this attachment. What beliefs do you hold about this person, thing, or situation that keep you attached? What healthy emotions and beliefs can you replace the unhealthy ones with?

Understand that this attachment not only causes you mental harm, but physical as well.

Tell yourself you are strong; you deserve to be happy and healthy in mind and body. Give yourself complete control over your life. You have given this person, thing, or feeling, power over you. They make you crazy, upset, angry, frustrated, or sad. It is time to take back that power and place it back within you where it belongs!

Be aware that the only person who can change your life is you. Everyone and everything else is out of your control. What others think, feel, how they act is not under your control. You cannot change them, but you can change the way you deal with them. When a difficult person or situation presents itself, see it and tell yourself that you'll let the Universe (or God) deal with it. Hand it over, move away from your need to change their behavior, and move on.

Continue to reinforce your detachment. You might feel as if you are slipping back into its hold, but just keep reinforcing the steps above. Remember the negative feelings that had a hold of you and how they made you feel; continue to replace them with positive feelings.[12]

Keep in mind that each emotion you experience is actually your soul speaking to you. Pay attention to what your soul is directing you to work on, as these are the lessons you came here to learn. You feel they manifested as a result of childhood, but in fact they came here in the form of your karma – these are the lessons you need to be working though.

You will also come to realize that certain people are in your life for certain reasons as part of your soul's learning process. For instance, the friend that enables you by reinforcing the false beliefs you hold. Or, the one who remains steadfast and true. Look back upon former relationships in which you had a choice to learn. From being used, to understanding false love, or by being abused. Did you learn something or did you to fail the

---

[12] How to Detach, page 35 of *BOOYAH! SPIRIT: 52 Ingredients for a Healthy Soul. Suffering is Optional.*, Sheila M. Burke, 2011, Om Sweet Om Publishing

test by failing to learn? Everyone in your life is there for some reason – *even if it seems minuscule.* They bring something with them into your energy that you will process internally and you will either learn from it, or not. If you learn you will nourish your soul; if you do not learn you will find these lessons popping back into your life.

Take a look at the things you experience over and over again in life. Maybe you feel like you never seem to progress (one step forward, two steps back), maybe you always seem to connect with people who are less than honest or don't have your best intentions at heart – whatever the issue is that you seem to constantly find yourself in – this is your cycle. You are experiencing this because this is what you are attracting. It is not the Universe conspiring against you – it is the Universe conspiring with you. Your soul is saying, "Bring me more of the same because I am failing to learn the lesson." Whether you are supposed to learn self-worth, patience, how to trust or be trusted, how to be honest, or any of the numerous lessons out there – there is a reason for the experience. You attract these people and situations because you have failed to learn in the past, and until you do learn, you will continue to be tested.

If you do not allow yourself to feel and experience your suffering, your pain, and your emotions; if you do not investigate the root of your suffering; if you do not talk about these issues – you will never break the cycle. You will remain trapped in your mind, telling yourself the same stories over and over again. You will become unable to move, afraid to trust your instincts, and you will remain paralyzed within your own suffering.

When it is a cyclical pattern you see repeated over and over again in yourself or your family – *these are not you.* You didn't come here with these patterns; this behavior is not a part of your true nature. You learned them by observation of your environment and those around you. You don't have to repeat them unless you want to repeat them. You have the ability to unlearn them, stop them, and go on with life in a healthy state. Trust your spirit and trust yourself, because within you, you actually have the answer to stop the cycle and the ability to do it!

When you allow yourself to feel, to put your energy and emotions under review and understand where they come from, to detach from all that is unhealthy, and work to make sure it sticks – it is at that point that you attract something different. This is your turning point. It is here that your once painful relationships can become healthy and flourish. It is here where you can say goodbye to suffering and hello to happiness. It is not until you are able to reach a place of peace that you will be able to move forward.

You have created the life you are living right now using action, words, and thought. Everything that has happened to you, everything you have lived in life, adds value to where you are headed. What you *do* with those experiences determines where you will go. If there is something different you would like to have, you must create something different.

Service to Others

When you are feeling down or out of sorts, when you are not sure of where you are at in this life – a place of solace can always be found through service to others. When you open your heart and share the love inside, you are guided to a place filled with hope, and the understanding that no matter where you are at right now – you can make a difference in the life of another. Through service to others we also serve our soul. When you reach out and extend your heart – when you freely give of your heart – you are opening up space within your heart for spirit to enter and fill it. The peace created within will give you a new found strength and the power to rise above your suffering.

Service to others gives us the ability to understand that we are all recovering from something; we are all working on our own issues. We are not alone, we are all in this together, have to be here for each other, and love each other. Everybody needs to take care of everybody else.

Make No Comparisons

Your journey is your journey. The biggest injustice you can do to your spirit is to compare your journey with someone else's journey. It might seem like some have it easier than you do; it may seem like some have it worse. The truth is – it doesn't matter because each of us have the same divine tools we need in order to make this journey, and they are all located within.

Your soul is following the path it needs to follow just like everyone else's soul is following their path. Your soul knew what it had to accomplish before it arrived here, and selected the road you are on now. Your soul placed confidence in its host – you. Now it is up to you to have confidence in your spirit, because it is divinely capable of leading you if you let it. Follow in your own footsteps.

You are not now, have never been, and will not ever be better than anyone or inferior to anyone. You are here at the Earth University to work on your soul. Make a decision right now, today, to break free from comparisons in order to become the student you were sent here to be.

10.

Synchronicity

There are no coincidences. *Not really.* They are actually signs – a nudge in the right direction. They appear when you have relaxed and opened your heart and mind to receiving a message or information, when you are ready to see things that you have simply not noticed before. When odd, serendipitous, or weird things happen it is because you have opened your heart and mind to receiving the message. You have put out there that you are ready – ready to learn, ready to see, and ready to discover. You have requested guidance and it is being delivered to you. You have ordered it up by thinking about it. You may feel goose-bumps and think of how weird that was, but actually it wasn't weird at all. It was a delicious platter of knowledge offered up to you from the Universe, from God, from a Higher Power.

When these things come to you, don't ignore them. Welcome them; see what they have to offer. When you are wondering about something and then suddenly start seeing signs everywhere that remind you of the thought – this means you need to put a little effort into the pursuit of that thought.

So, the next time you think you are experiencing one of life's "coincidences" – it's actually a tap on your shoulder meant to get you to stop and pay attention. It's an illumination of the path ahead to a place where you might find something you are looking for, or it may lead you to somewhere you may need to be. Much in the same way that you can look up at the clear night sky and see millions of stars but not see every one of them, or not see all the movement up there – our minds are processing millions of things constantly. Our brains know what we are thinking about most often, what's bugging us, what's making us happy, and it is therefore screening our thoughts for more of the same to let our mind chew on. When we are able to quiet our mind, the flood of thoughts, we are able to make space for thoughts that would normally be thrown out by our screening brain. We create a calm and hospitable environment to invite those thoughts inside.

Coincidences are in fact your soul's way of summoning up something it needs from the Universe. A piece of the puzzle that just might help you along your way, take you to somewhere or someone you had trouble locating, and aid your journey.

"There are no coincidences.
It is your soul whispering to you in dreams,
during waking hours, and in quiet moments.
Leading you; shining for you;
a beacon home"
Sheila Burke

11.

Teach The Children Well

As a mom I understand the importance of raising children to be strong and happy. I also understand that it takes more than just the parent to raise, or influence, the child. It truly does take a village to raise a child. Children learn from everyone they are in contact with, so it is our divine duty to display and convey to them the very best we have within ourselves. To see peace and love prevail on earth, we must first find these things ourselves – and then we must teach them to our children. By *our children*, I mean all of our children, even if we are not their natural parents.

Let's teach our children the importance of inner being, a healthy inner self, and inner peace. Teach them the value of personal space and following their heart; instruct them on honesty and the importance of chasing dreams. Educate them with patience and soft guidance. Help them to understand that mistakes happen and consequences are a part of growth.

Teach them to value their own opinion and how to dare to be different. Teach them to say no in uncomfortable situations and to weigh possible outcomes before decision making. Let them make their own mistakes, and encourage them, without judgment, to find their way back when they lose their way. Always leave the proverbial light on for them. Instill in your child the fact that they do not have to be overcome by anger, fear, jealousy, greed or negative emotion – that it is okay to experience these things, but it is unhealthy to hold on to them.

Teach them to believe in themselves, trust their intuition, and to think for themselves. Be patient with them. Tell them you are proud of them. We all know that when a child is in the room, they can hear everything – even when you think they are not paying attention. Think before you act and speak – someone very impressionable is watching and listening. Last but not least, our children tend to react as we react; they take our cues and develop the same patterns as we have. Therefore, there is no better time than the present to make some changes for the better in your own life – not only for your sake, but for the sake of the child.

Encourage the love of nature, spend time outside, let them absorb and experience wonder. Teach them we are all a part of nature and that nature can help us relax and heal our spirit. Share your awakened heart by being a beacon to a child who is lost in darkness.

12.

The Answers to Life's Questions

The feeling of awakening is a real rush. A rush of excitement within – you can literally feel energy pulsing throughout your body. Life feels wonderful and amazing. It's as if you can see life from the perspective of outside yourself, watching your own thoughts unfold. Divine love encompasses you and in that moment the world seems to make complete sense. You see love everywhere, in everyone, and in everything. It's a feeling you could easily settle into for the duration of your life. *If it were possible, that is.* I mean, I'm sure it's possible, but for the majority of us it is not possible to remain within that place for long without really working on it constantly.

Awakening doesn't mean you will never hurt again; it doesn't mean you will continue to remain in that state of mind. It does, however, mean that you have found, or are on track to find, the tools within you to return to that state when you need too. It's a feeling that cannot be totally described yet is one of the most beautiful you will ever feel. It is *home*.

Do as much as you can within your living years to facilitate the transition of your soul in your dying days. Remember, everything imprints upon your soul and lessons not learned will be repeated. We have entered this life as part of our journey to become Divine. All the external junk that we process and worry about every day is wasting our precious time at Earth U. Take the time to understand, practice and live through this guide to awakening.

When your soul gets sick, and it will every now and then, take the time and energy to understand where it is coming from and then fix it. You have the tools and the power inside you, your Sacred Seed, to work through all the issues you have and live a life to nourish your soul. The amazing feeling you experience when everything feels good and right – is your soul communicating directly to you. Do more of that; do more of what makes your soul sing.

We are here to become rich. Not monetarily, but rich in love, rich in compassion, and rich in understanding. We are here to become abundant of spirit. There are so many beautiful things on this planet that we generally don't pay attention to. We walk by them without giving them a second thought. From the clouds floating in the afternoon sky to the vibrant colors of an autumn day –

leaves once green and perched upon a branch up high, now rest upon the earth.

Those who experience awakening have learned to drape the human experience around them like a fluffy blanket on a cool night. Not the human experience of the rat race, the 9-5 job, or problems of everyday life – we have learned to process our experience in a much different way. We seek and find the absolute pure beauty within nature; we are fully aware of the spiritual importance of giving of ourselves to others; we see the small things are actually the big picture. It is not that we never experience that big hamster wheel of human existence – the daily grind; we simply understand that none of that matters in relation to the purpose of why we are here in the first place. We are comforted in a space of love, compassion, and appreciation for all. We admire what has gone into the creation of life and find wonder and amazement in the ability to see it in detail.

What happens when we strip away every "thing" from our lives: gender, occupation, bills, beauty, race, ethnicity, our role in life, social status, political parties, our fears, our problems? Everything we *think* we are – put it all aside. *What remains?* We are left with our pure and authentic self. Pure consciousness that cares absolutely nothing about any of those other humanly layers. Pure consciousness that is here to cultivate its place in a divine realm using love, empathy, and an open heart – through compassion, grace, patience, and appreciation for all that is – *including the ugly bits.*

When I die it will not matter what political party I supported, what I did for a living, or how much money I made. It won't matter in the least. What will matter is how well I loved from my heart – *how well I loved everyone*, not just the nice people; it will matter how I treated other living beings; it will matter how I appreciated all living things and how much of myself I was willing to share with others. It will matter how much respected life in every aspect and all that went into the creation of it.

Live one day at a time. Take the hints of today and follow them. Pray, meditate, clear your mind; persevere; be confident. Love yourself as you are right now. You are strong, beautiful, and amazing. You have the power within your soul to get through whatever obstacles are in your way.

Life is speaking to you. You may not always like what it's saying, but you still have to listen. Find the lesson in the day. You are not perfect and will never be perfect. Once you come to terms that you are who you are at this moment – no more, no less – *and you appreciate all you have right now* – you *will* blossom.

Spiritual awakening is living life through your whole being; living life through love, not fear. By living the life you choose to live, you become what you are. *You create your own reality.* Enjoy who you are – *every single part of you.*

Who am I?

You are pure, divine consciousness; you are a member of the Chorus of Souls. You possess the wisdom of the Universe.

Why am I here?

You are in human form to learn by experiencing; to teach with love. Your quest is Divine growth through compassion, grace, patience, and unconditional love.

Where am I going?

Eventually, you will return to Source, but not before you have learned all you need to learn – through life, death, and rebirth.

How do I grow?

Soul growth begins with loving who you are, right now at this moment, *no matter what place you are in.* It is never too early, and it is certainly never too late to do what you love, to change your life, or awaken gifts within your soul. Follow your intuition, your heart. It may not always seem as if the path you're led to is the direct path, but it is leading you through to the learning experience that your soul needs. Pay attention to the signs – to what your soul is telling you. Follow the practices of healing a sick soul and maintain the cultivation for a healthy spiritual practice. There is no greater gift you can give your soul than to love all living beings. Too see the divine love and light behind all eyes, *behind all life*, regardless of circumstance or appearance. **Be Love**.

Namaste

I respect the place in you that is of love,
of truth, and of Light ~
your Spirit; your Soul;
where divinity is; where God resides.
When you are in that place within you,
and I am in that place within me,
our minds meet and we are one.

Sheila M. Burke

About the Author

Sheila Burke was born and raised in Northeast Ohio. In 1989 she married her soul mate Shane, and together they have delighted in raising their three beautiful children into strong young adults.

Always a dabbler in putting pen to paper, Burke finally started publishing her books in 2010 with the release of her first book *Zen-Sational Living*. Her journey of self-discovery started after getting over the hurdle of raising teenagers without losing all of her marbles. Learning how to live a life where stress takes a backseat and love rides shotgun is reflected in her writing. She shares her knowledge of spirit and soul, of all she understands, freely and simply through her many titles.

Other Books by Sheila Burke

(available at bookstores)

Zen-Sational Living:
A Simple Guide to Finding Your True Self and Maintaining Balance

Loaded with sensible advice, Zen-Sational Living is a road-map for making good decisions and being your best. From the basics of Zen, to health (mental and physical), creating a personal space, and everything in between! Whether you're in need of a boost, a change, or are starting on your own road of self-discovery, ZEN-SATIONAL LIVING will guide you on your journey. With easy to follow chapters on judgment, focus, compassion, forgiveness, stress, relaxation, and many more; Burke guides the reader in making simple, mindful adjustments for a healthier spirit, mind, and body. This book is truly an amazing guide on how to appreciate life and enjoy life.

Booyah! Spirit:
52 Ingredients for a Healthy Soul. Suffering Is Optional

BOOYAH! SPIRIT merges scientific research, humor, wonderful pictures, quotes, how-tos, and personal life lessons to help you live the life of your dreams. The expression "Booyah" is one that many people would yell after one performs a difficult feat. But I also discovered that Booyah "is a food that is prepared like a stew, but on a very large scale. It takes many cooks to prepare the food, and it is usually meant to serve hundreds or even thousands of people". Not unlike Booyah Stew, this book is filled with ideas to nourish the souls of hundreds or even thousands of people. BOOYAH! SPIRIT combines ancient ideas with new ones. There are 52 chapters that represent the weeks of the year.

Circle of Soul: at the end, we begin again

CIRCLE OF SOUL guides the reader through finding their inner Spirit - a place that for many has become lost over time through the rigors of everyday life. Sages throughout the ages have taught us how to live a spiritual life - it is not a secret. A personal journey doesn't have to be difficult, this book will help you get started and on your way.

Whispers of the Soul

WHISPERS OF THE SOUL is the 5th title released by inspirational author Sheila M. Burke. Whispers is a full color poster book filled with original photography and original quotes from the author about the soul, soul mates, and soul connections.

Did you ever meet someone and become fast friends, where you feel as if you have known them your entire life, although you've only just met recently? I know those feelings well; I have them on occasion. I think they are leftover energies, imprints if you will, left upon the universe from times past. A wink and smile and perhaps a bond from another time that went deep. Coming full circle and finding you again in this lifetime.

150 Ways to Get Your Zen On:
Book 1 – Finding Your Happy Place

150 Ways to Get Your Zen On:
Book 2 – Simple Pleasures

It's the simple things we do or enjoy daily that help us find our Zen. Belly laughs, the warmth of a sunrise, kindness, puppy kisses, or thick, fuzzy socks. The little things that help you to relax and let all the stress slide off your shoulders.

These books provide 150 examples each of simple thinking designed to help you find your happy place. Zen is not about never feeling sad, angry, joyful, or having fun; Zen is the understanding that by not clinging (or attaching) ourselves to these feelings, we can free ourselves from them and enjoy life to the fullest.

www.SheilaMBurke.com   **facebook.com/BeZensational**

www.ingramcontent.com/pod-product-compliance
Lightning Source LLC
Chambersburg PA
CBHW050131280326
41933CB00010B/1330